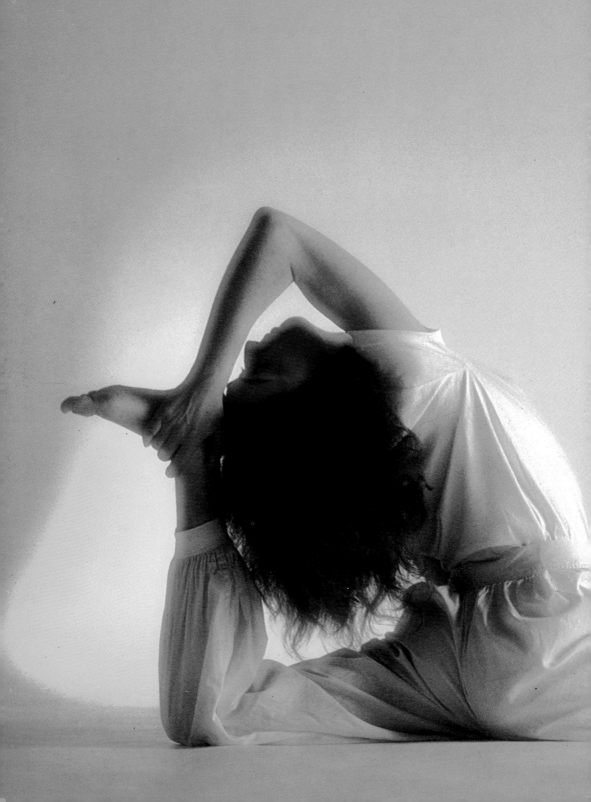

THE SIVANANDA COMPANION TO
YOGA

Foreword by Swami Vishnu Devananda

Written by Lucy Lidell
with Narayani and Giris Rabinovitch
Photography by Fausto Dorelli

A GAIA ORIGINAL

A Fireside Book
Published by Simon & Schuster Inc.
New York   London   Toronto   Sydney   Tokyo

A GAIA ORIGINAL

Written by Lucy Lidell
with Narayani and Giris Rabinovitch
Photography by Fausto Dorelli

from an idea by
Lucy Lidell

Direction	Joss Pearson
	Patrick Nugent
Editorial	Roslin Mair
Design	Tony Spalding
	Chris Meehan
	David Whelan
	Sheilagh Noble

A Fireside Book
Published by Simon & Schuster Inc.
Simon & Schuster Building, Rockefeller Center,
1230 Avenue of the Americas, New York, New York 10020
FIRESIDE and colophon are registered trademarks of Simon and Schuster, Inc.

Printed in Spain by Artes Graficas Toledo, S.A.

7 9 8 6

Library of Congress Cataloging in Publication Data
Main entry under title:
The Sivananda companion to yoga.
  includes index.
  1. Yoga, Hatha.
RA781.7.S584 1983   613.7'046.   83-9398
ISBN 0-671-47088-4

D.L.TO: 1423–1989

To Swami Vishnu Devananda

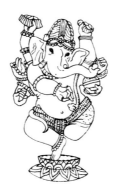

How to Use this Book

This book gives you all the information you will need to begin to practise yoga at home. The core of your practice is laid down in *The Basic Session*. There is a simple chart on pages 66-67 showing the beginner how to proceed, and in *The Cycle of Life* you will find modified practice sessions for particular physical conditions and ages – notably Pregnancy and the Later Years.

Use the Basic Session for constant reference as you add in to your session the *Relaxation* and *Breathing* techniques. Once you are familiar with the Basic Session, and simple breathing and meditation practices, you can begin to add in the material given in *Asanas and Variations,* and more advanced breathing and meditation. By working in this way you should build up a regular daily routine that suits your lifestyle. Do go to yoga classes as well, as this will enhance your own practice sessions.

NOTE It is important that you follow the directions step-by-step, finding your own pace, and proceed systematically according to the advice given on the order of asanas, the relaxation periods, and the length of practice. Always observe any cautions and never strain in a pose. There is no need to rush or force yourself – all bodies are different and you will find your own level naturally.

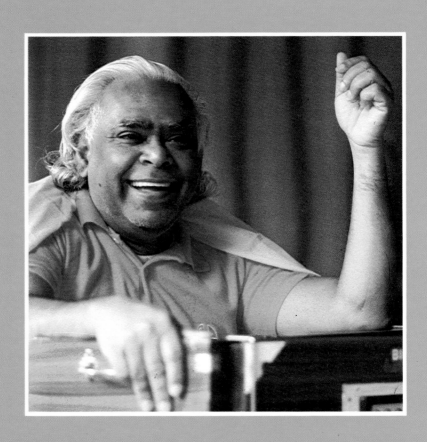

Foreword

Today, more than at any other time in the history of humanity, people in the West are facing stresses and tensions that are beyond their control. Thousands and thousands are turning to tranquillizers, sleeping pills, alcohol and so on in a vain attempt to cope. In 1957 I arrived in America, sent by my Master, Swami Sivananda. My Master said: "Go, people are waiting. Many souls from the East are reincarnating now in the West. Go and reawaken the consciousness hidden in their memories and bring them back to the path of Yoga."

Yoga, the oldest science of life, can teach you to bring stress under control – not only on a physical level, but on mental and spiritual levels too. The human body can be compared to a car. There are five things that any automobile needs to run properly, whether it is a Rolls Royce or a rusty old car – lubrication, a cooling system, electric current, fuel and a sensible driver behind the wheel. In Yoga, the asanas or postures lubricate the body. They keep the muscles and joints running smoothly, tone all the internal organs, and increase circulation, without creating any fatigue. The body is cooled by complete relaxation whilst pranayama or yogic breathing increases prana, the electric current. Fuel is provided by food, water and the air you breathe. Lastly, you have meditation which stills the mind, the driver of the body. By meditating, you learn to control and ultimately transcend the body – your physical vehicle.

Anyone can practise Yoga, no matter what their age, condition or religion. Young or old, sick or fit, – all can benefit from this discipline. After all, everyone has to breathe, whatever their walk of life. And we all get arthritis if we eat the wrong food. You can learn to meditate on a flower, the Star of David or the Cross just as well as on Krishna or Rama. The object of concentration can be different but the technique remains the same. The first yogis sought answers to two fundamental questions – "How can I get rid of pain?" and "How can I conquer death?" They discovered that through asanas you can control the physical pain, through pranayama the emotional pain, and through meditation you can come to a real understanding of who you are. Free from false identification with name and form, you can transcend the body altogether and find the Self which is immortal. So you see, though Yoga begins with the body it ends by transcending it.

In conclusion, I would like to tell you all that Yoga is not a theory but a practical way of life. If you have never tasted honey, no matter how often I tell you that honey is good you won't understand until you try it. Put Yoga into practice and you will see the benefit for yourself. This book will help you to get started, and serve as a companion and inspiration along the way.

Swami Vishnudevananda

Contents

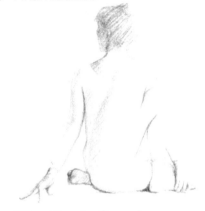

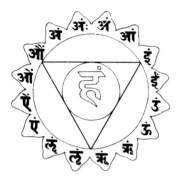

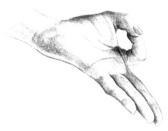

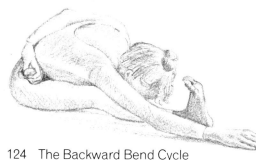

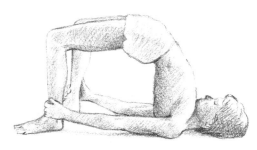

156 The Cycle of Life

176 Yoga and Health

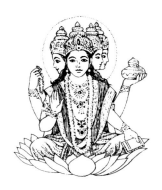

Introduction to Yoga

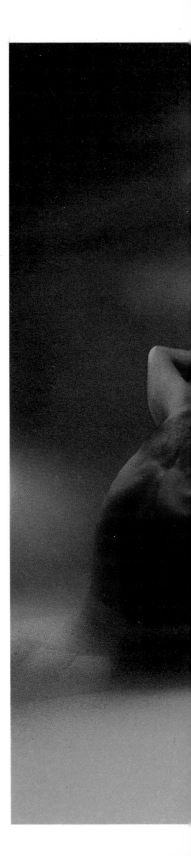

Anyone can practise yoga. You don't need special equipment or clothes – just a small amount of space and a strong desire for a healthier, more fulfilled life. The yoga postures or asanas exercise every part of the body, stretching and toning the muscles and joints, the spine and the entire skeletal system. And they work not only on the body's frame but on the internal organs, glands and nerves as well, keeping all systems in radiant health. By releasing physical and mental tension, they also liberate vast resources of energy. The yogic breathing exercises known as pranayama revitalize the body and help to control the mind, leaving you feeling calm and refreshed, while the practice of positive thinking and meditation gives increased clarity, mental power and concentration.

Yoga is a complete science of life that originated in India many thousands of years ago. It is the oldest system of personal development in the world, encompassing body, mind and spirit. The ancient yogis had a profound understanding of man's essential nature and of what he needs to live in harmony with himself and his environment. They perceived the physical body as a vehicle, with the mind as the driver, the soul man's true identity, and action, emotion and intelligence as the three forces which pull the body-vehicle. In order for there to be integrated development these three forces must be in balance. Taking into account the interrelationship between body and mind, they formulated a unique method for maintaining this balance – a method that combines all the movements you need for physical health with the breathing and meditation techniques that ensure peace of mind.

Yoga in your Life

Many people are first drawn to yoga as a way to keep their bodies fit and supple – good to look at and to live in. Others come seeking help or relief for a specific complaint, like tension or backache. Some are merely impelled by a sense that they are not getting as much out of life as they could be. Whatever your reason, yoga can be a tool, an instrument for you – giving you both what you came for, and more. To understand what yoga is all about you need to experience it for yourself. At first glance it seems to be little more than a series of strange physical postures, which keep the body lean and flexible. But in time, anyone who continues with regular practice becomes aware of a subtle change in their approach to life – for, through persistently toning and relaxing the body and stilling the mind, you begin to glimpse a state of inner peace which is your true nature. It is this that constitutes the essence of yoga – this self-realization that we are all seeking, consciously or unconsciously, and towards which we are all gradually evolving.

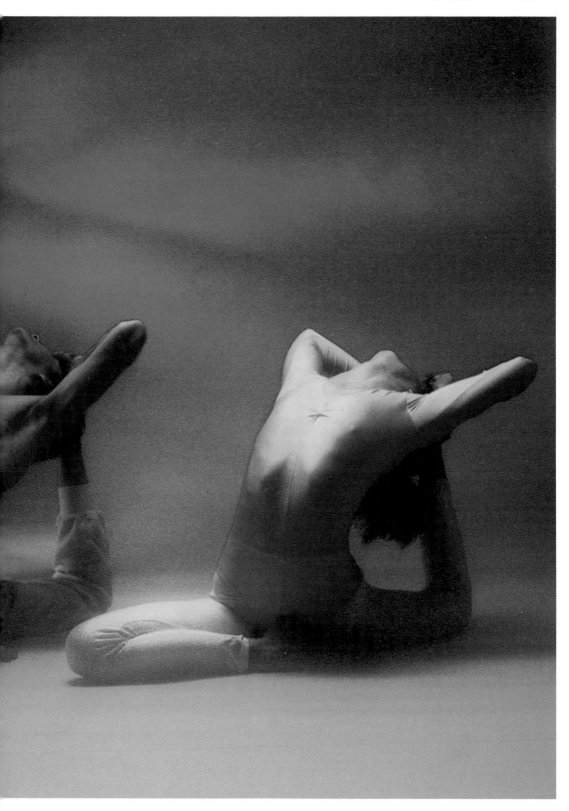

If you can bring your mind and thoughts under control, there is literally no limit to what you can do – since it is only our own illusions and preconceptions that hold us back and prevent us from fulfilling ourselves.

The Physiology of Yoga

Just as we expect our cars to depreciate in value with age, so we resign ourselves to the fact that our bodies will function less efficiently with the passing years – never stopping to ask ourselves if this is really necessary, or why it is that animals seem able to go on functioning well throughout most of their lives, while we do not. In fact, ageing is largely an artificial condition, caused mainly by auto-intoxication or self-poisoning. Through keeping the body parts clean and well-lubricated, we can significantly reduce the catabolic process of cell deterioration.

In recent years, medical research has begun to pay attention to the effects of yoga. Studies have shown, for instance, that relaxation in the Corpse Pose effectively relieves high blood pressure and that regular practice of asanas and pranayama can help such diverse ailments as arthritis, arteriosclerosis, chronic fatigue, asthma, varicose veins and heart conditions. Laboratory tests have also confirmed yogis' ability to consciously control autonomic or involuntary functions, such as temperature, heartbeat and blood pressure. One study of the effects of Hatha Yoga over six months demonstrated the following effects: significantly increased

Imprints of Energy
The energizing effect of the yoga postures or asanas is clearly revealed by the Kirlian photographs shown below. The imprint on the left was taken before a 15-minute session of asanas. When the same subject's hand was rephotographed after the session, a fuller, more complete aura was revealed. Interestingly, a 15-minute session of gymnastics with the same subject failed to produce any change in aura.

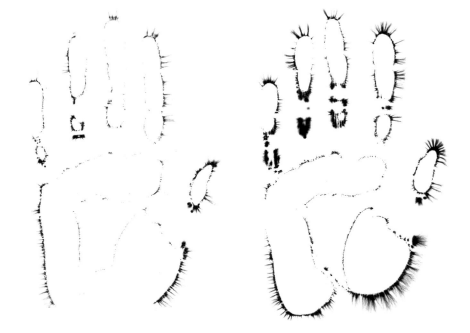

lung capacity and respiration; reduced body weight and girth; an improved ability to resist stress; and a decrease in cholesterol and blood sugar level – all resulting in a stabilizing and restorative effect on the body's natural systems. Today there can no longer be any doubt of yoga's effectiveness as both a curative and preventive medicine.

The History of Yoga

The origins of yoga are shrouded in the mists of time – for yoga is regarded as a divine science of life, revealed to enlightened sages in meditation. The oldest archaeological evidence of its existence is provided by a number of stone seals showing figures in yogic postures, excavated from the Indus valley and thought to date from around 3000 BC. Yoga is first mentioned in the vast collection of scriptures called the Vedas, portions of which date from at least 2500 BC, but it is the Upanishads, which form the later part of the Vedas, that provide the main foundation of yoga teaching, and of the philosophy known as Vedanta. Central to Vedanta is the idea of one absolute reality or consciousness, known as Brahman, that underlies the entire universe.

Around the sixth century BC appeared two massive epic poems – the Ramayana, written by Valmiki, and the Mahabharata, written by Vyasa and containing the Bhagavad Gita, perhaps the best known of all yogic scriptures. In the Gita, God or Brahman, incarnated as Lord Krishna, instructs the warrior Arjuna in yoga – specifically in how to achieve

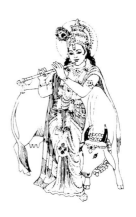

Krishna

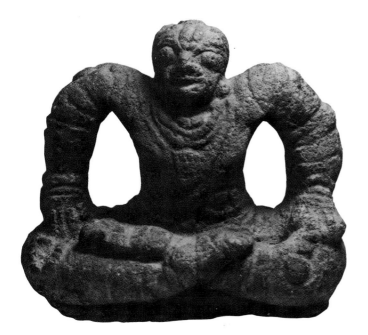

Meditating Yogi
Evidence of the ancient lineage of yoga is provided by numerous paintings and carvings of the practice. This small medieval stone statue shows a yogi in the Lotus Pose.

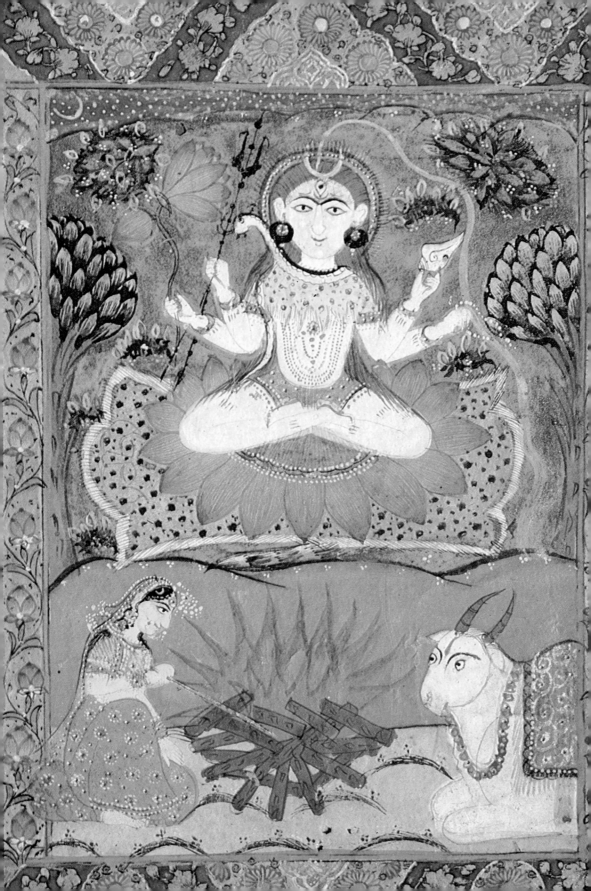

liberation by fulfilling one's duties in life. The backbone of Raja Yoga is furnished by Patanjali's Yoga Sutras (p.19), thought to have been written in the third century BC. The classical text on Hatha Yoga is the Hatha Yoga Pradipika, which describes the various asanas and breathing exercises which form the basis of the modern practice of yoga.

"The bow is the sacred OM and the arrow is our own soul. Brahman is the mark of the arrow, the aim of the soul. Even as an arrow becomes one with its mark, let the watchful soul be one in him."
Mundaka Upanishad

The Meaning of Yoga

The underlying purpose of all the different aspects of the practice of yoga is to reunite the individual self (jiva) with the Absolute or pure consciousness (Brahman) – in fact, the word yoga means literally "joining". Union with this unchanging reality liberates the spirit from all sense of separation, freeing it from the illusion of time, space and causation. It is only our own ignorance, our inability to discriminate between the real and unreal, that prevents us from realizing our true nature.

Even in this ignorance, the human spirit often perceives that something is lacking in life – something that neither achieving

Traditionally, the god Siva is regarded as the original founder of Yoga.

India's temporal rulers have always sought the spiritual wisdom of the yogis.

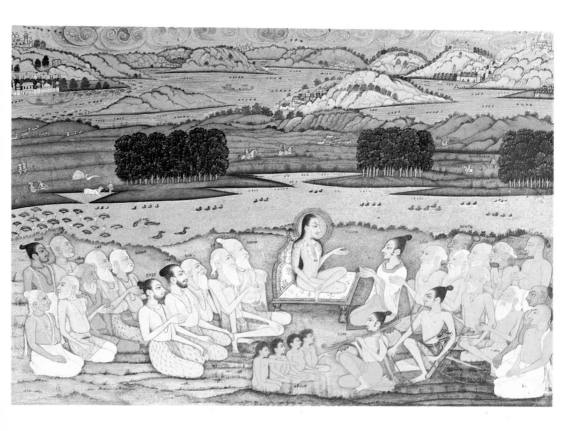

a goal nor fulfilling a desire can satisfy. In each individual life, the restless search for love, for success, for change, for happiness are all witness to this underlying awareness of a reality we sense but cannot reach.

In yoga teaching, reality is by definition unchanging and unmoving – the world, the manifest universe, which is in a perpetual state of flux is therefore illusion, or Maya. This is symbolised in the image of Siva, Lord of the Dance, depicted with his foot raised – when he puts his foot down, the universe as we know it will cease to exist. The manifest universe is only a superimposition on the real, it is projected on the screen of reality, much as a movie is projected on a screen at the cinema. Just as, walking in the dark, we may mistake a piece of rope for a snake, so without illumination we mistake the unreal for the real – we superimpose or project our own illusions on the real world.

The illusory nature of temporal reality is reflected in the search of modern science for the ultimate, indivisible particle of matter. This has led to the realisation that matter and energy are interchangeable, that the semblance of solidity we perceive in matter is created by movement or vibration – we see a moving fan as a whole circle. Most of what we perceive as solid is in fact empty space; if we were to take away all the space from all the atoms in our bodies, retaining only the "non-space", we would not even be able to see what was left.

The Creation of Maya

In yoga philosophy, there was originally only the Self – undifferentiated energy, infinite, unchanging and formless. The process of differentiation which has led to the manifest universe, the physical world we know, is described in several different ways. First there was the Spirit, or Purusha; then came a great light (the "big bang" theory) which caused the evolution of the objective universe, as Prakriti, the manifest world we perceive. Once Prakriti moved out, the three qualities known as gunas (p.80) were differentiated, whereas in Purusha they were in equilibrium. The same process is sometimes described as the differentiation of "I" and "this", of subject and object , and mythologically as Shakti moving out from Siva – in the raising of Kundalini (p.70), when the state of superconsciousness is attained, the two principles are reunited and the illusion is no more.

Karma and Reincarnation

To a yogi, body and mind are part of the illusory world of matter, with a limited life span, but the spirit is eternal and passes on when one body wears out, to another. As the Bhagavad Gita says: "Just as a man casts off worn-out clothes and puts on new ones, so also the embodied Self casts off worn-out bodies and enters others which are new." Through

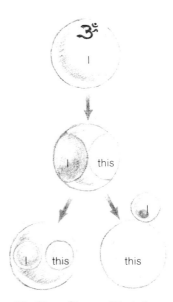

The Three Stages of Evolution
In the diagram above "I" represents oneness and "this", matter. Before evolution, all is one, prana is in a potential state. In the intermediate stage, prana becomes active, creating matter – still perceived as part of the oneness. In the last stage – the manifest universe – there are two steps: first, matter is perceived as separate from the oneness (left); second, both mind and matter are perceived as separate from the oneness (right).

The Yogi and the Peacock
This eighteenth-century print de- picts a yogi feeding a peacock as a form of devotion – in Hindu mythology, the peacock repre- sents Krishna.

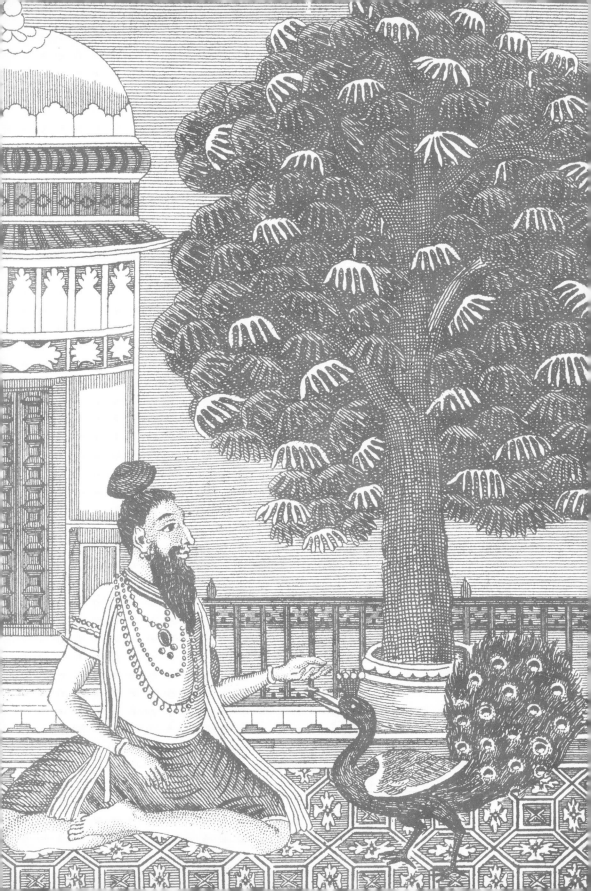

the cycle of reincarnation, we draw nearer to reuniting with the Self within, as the veil of ignorance grows thinner. Central to yogic thought is the law of Karma – of cause and effect, action and reaction. Every action and thought bear fruit – whether in this life or in future lives. We reap what we sow, moulding our future by what we do and think in the present.

The Paths of Yoga

There are four main paths of yoga – Karma Yoga, Bhakti Yoga, Jnana Yoga and Raja Yoga. Each suited to a different temperament or approach to life. All the paths lead ultimately to the same destination – to union with Brahman or God – and the lessons of each of them need to be integrated if true wisdom is to be attained. Karma Yoga – the yoga of action – is

The Wheel of Life and Death
The wheel symbolizes the cycle of existence – the perpetual cycle of birth, death and rebirth, from which man is liberated when he achieves Self-realization.

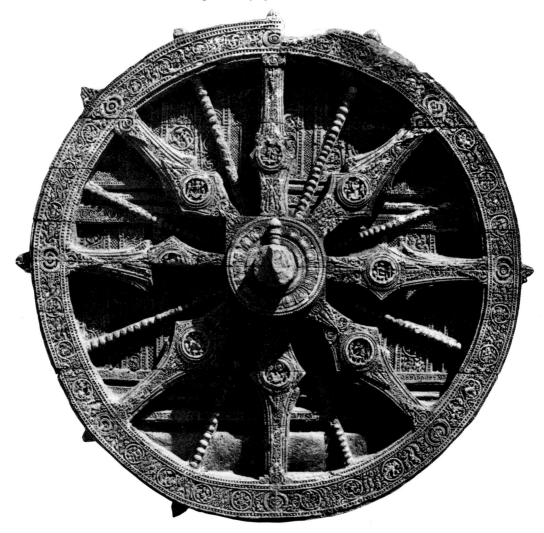

the path chosen primarily by those of an outgoing nature. It purifies the heart by teaching you to act selflessly, without thought of gain or reward. By detaching yourself from the fruits of your actions and offering them up to God, you learn to sublimate the ego. To achieve this, it is helpful to keep your mind focused by repeating a mantra (p.99) while engaged in any activity. Bhakti Yoga is the path of devotion, which appeals particularly to those of an emotional nature. The Bhakti yogi is motivated chiefly by the power of love and sees God as the embodiment of love. Through prayer, worship and ritual he surrenders himself to God, channelling and trans-muting his emotions into unconditional love or devotion. Chanting or singing the praises of God form a substantial part of Bhakti Yoga. Jnana Yoga – the yoga of knowledge or wisdom – is the most difficult path, requiring tremendous strength of will and intellect. Taking the philosophy of Vedanta the Jnana yogi uses his mind to inquire into its own nature. We perceive the space inside and outside a glass as different, just as we see ourselves as separate from God. Jnana Yoga leads the devotee to experience his unity with God directly by breaking the glass, dissolving the veils of ignorance. Before practising Jnana Yoga, the aspirant needs to have integrated the lessons of the other yogic paths – for without selflessness and love of God, strength of body and mind, the search for self-realization can become mere idle speculation. Raja Yoga – the path we deal with chiefly in this book – is the science of physical and mental control. Often called the "royal road" it offers a comprehensive method for controlling the waves of thought by turning our mental and physical energy into spiritual energy.

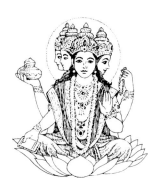

Brahma

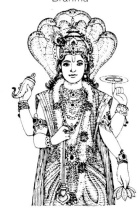

Vishnu

The Eight Limbs of Raja Yoga

Compiled by the Sage Patanjali in the Yoga Sutras, the Eight Limbs are a progressive series of steps or disciplines which purify the body and mind, ultimately leading the yogi to enlightenment: yamas; niyamas; asanas; pranayama; praty-ahara; dharana; dhyana; and samadhi. The yamas or restraints are divided into five moral injunctions, aimed at destroying the lower nature: non-violence; truthfulness in word, thought and deed; non-stealing; moderation in all things; and non-possessiveness. The niyamas or observances are also divided into five. Fostering positive qualities, they consist of: purity; contentment; austerity; study of the sacred texts; and constantly living with an awareness of the Divine Presence. Asanas or postures and pranayama – regulation of breath – form the sub-division of Raja Yoga known as Hatha Yoga. Pratyahara means drawing the senses inward in order to still the mind, in preparation for dharana or concentration. Dharana leads to dhyana or meditation, culminating in samadhi or superconsciousness,

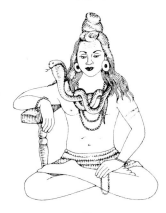

Siva

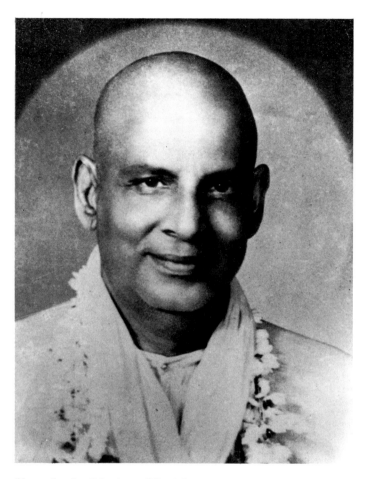

H. H. Sri Swami Sivananda
Born in 1887, Swami Sivananda was a great yogi and sage who devoted his life to the service of humanity and the study of Vedanta. His prescription for a spiritual life is summed up in six simple commands: "Serve. Love. Give. Purify. Meditate. Realise."

Yoga in the Modern World

Yoga is a living science – one that has evolved over thousands of years and continues to evolve in accordance with the needs of humanity. One of the most important figures in its recent development has been Swami Sivananda. This great Indian master trained and worked as a doctor before renouncing the world for the spiritual path. A man of prodigious energy and strength, he published over 300 books, pamphlets and journals, bringing the authority of his medical background to bear on the teachings of yoga, while explaining the most complex philosophical subjects in simple, straightforward terms. Besides establishing an Ashram and a Yoga Academy, Sivananda founded the Divine Life Society in 1935, dedicated to the ideals of truth, purity, non-violence and self-realization. At his Ashram in Rishikesh, he trained many exceptional disciples in yoga and Vedanta – among them, Swami Vishnu Devananda, whom he sent to spread the practice of yoga in the West. Swami Vishnu arrived in San Francisco in 1957 and

The Five Principles

Proper Relaxation *releases tension in the muscles and rests the whole system, leaving you as refreshed as after a good night's sleep. It carries over into all your activities and teaches you to conserve your energy and let go of all worries or fears.*

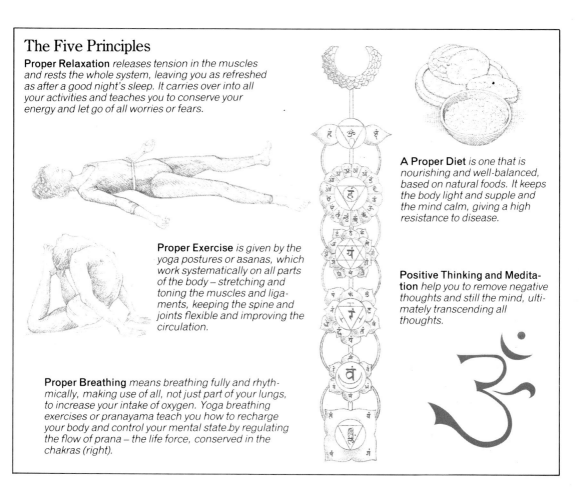

Proper Exercise *is given by the yoga postures or asanas, which work systematically on all parts of the body – stretching and toning the muscles and ligaments, keeping the spine and joints flexible and improving the circulation.*

Proper Breathing *means breathing fully and rhythmically, making use of all, not just part of your lungs, to increase your intake of oxygen. Yoga breathing exercises or pranayama teach you how to recharge your body and control your mental state by regulating the flow of prana – the life force, conserved in the chakras (right).*

A Proper Diet *is one that is nourishing and well-balanced, based on natural foods. It keeps the body light and supple and the mind calm, giving a high resistance to disease.*

Positive Thinking and Meditation *help you to remove negative thoughts and still the mind, ultimately transcending all thoughts.*

travelled for several years throughout the United States, lecturing and demonstrating asanas, before establishing an international network of Sivananda Yoga Centres and Ashrams. As well as being one of the foremost exponents of Raja and Hatha Yoga in the world, Swami Vishnu is also actively dedicated to the cause of peace and universal brotherhood – on one of his peace missions in 1971, he piloted a small plane to the troublespots of the world – Belfast, the Suez Canal, and Lahore, West Pakistan – "bombarding" them with leaflets calling for an end to violence. A teacher of great personal dynamism, Swami Vishnu has inspired thousands of students at his Ashrams and changed the lives of many more through his writings. By closely observing the lifestyles and needs of people in the West, he has synthesized the ancient wisdom of yoga into five basic principles that can easily be incorporated into your own pattern of living, to provide the foundation of a long and healthy life. It is around these five principles – summarized above – that this book is structured.

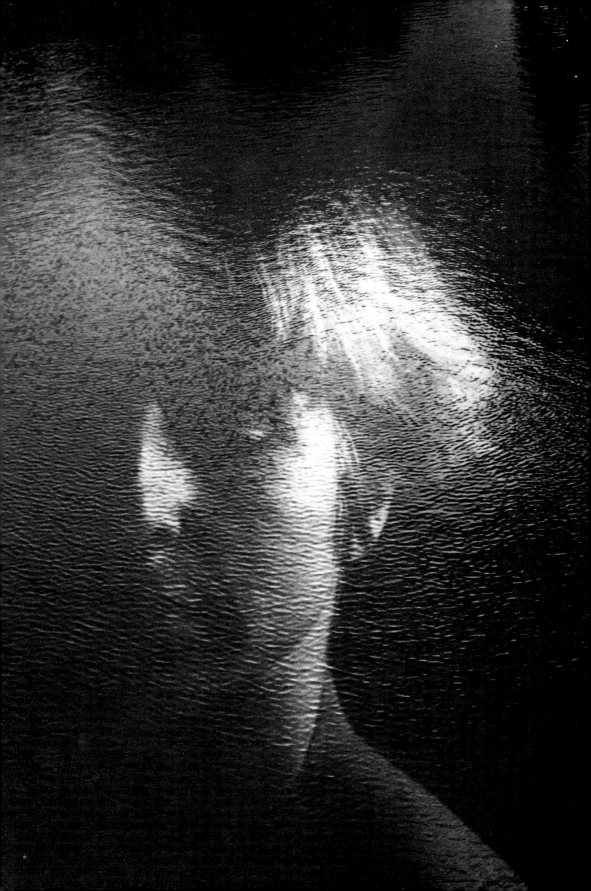

Relaxation

*"The soul that moves in the world of
the senses and yet keeps the senses in
harmony . . . finds rest in quietness."*
Bhagavad Gita

Living with mind and body relaxed is our natural state, our birthright – it is only the pace of our lives that has made us forget. Those who retain the art possess the key to good health, vitality and peace of mind, for relaxation is a tonic for the whole being, liber- ating vast resources of energy.

The state of our minds and the state of our bodies are intimately linked. If your muscles are relaxed, then your mind must be relaxed. If the mind is anxious, then the body suffers too. All action originates in the mind. When the mind receives a stimulus that alerts it to the need for action, it sends a message via the nerves to contract the muscles in readi- ness. In the hustle and bustle of the modern world, the mind is continuously bombarded with stimuli which may cause us to freeze in the alerted "fight or flight" pattern of re- sponse. As a result, many people spend much of their lives – even while asleep – in a state of physical and mental tension. Every- one has their own particular trouble spots – whether it is a clenched jaw, a furrowed brow, or a stiff neck. This unnecessary tension not only causes a lot of discomfort but is an enormous drain on our energy resources and a major cause of tiredness and ill-health. For energy is being used both to tell the muscles to contract and to keep them contracted, even if we are only half aware of it.

In this section we present the technique of relaxation that is an essential part of your yoga practice. There are three parts to proper relaxation – physical, mental and spiritual relaxation. To relax the body, you lie down in the Corpse Pose (p.24) and first tense then relax each part of the body in turn, working up from your feet to your head. This alternate tensing then relaxing is necessary because it

is only by knowing how tension feels that you can be sure that you have achieved relaxation. Then, just as in normal life your mind in- structs the muscles to tense and contract, you now use autosuggestion to send the muscles a message to relax. With practice you will gradually learn to use your subconscious mind to extend this control to the involuntary muscles of the heart, the digestive systems and other organs too.

To relax and focus the mind you breathe steadily and rhymthmically and concentrate on your breathing. Mental and physical re- laxation can never be complete, however, until you achieve spiritual peace. For as long as you identify with your body and mind, there will be fears and worries, anger and sorrow. Spiritual relaxation means detaching yourself, becoming a witness of the body and mind in order to identify with the Self or pure con- sciousness – the source of truth and peace that lies within us all.

As you relax, you will feel sensations of melting down, of expansion, lightness and warmth. When all muscular tension is gone, a gentle euphoria suffuses the whole body. Relaxation is not so much a state as a process, a series of levels of increasing depth. It is a matter of letting go, instead of holding on; of not doing, rather than doing. As you relax the whole body and breathe slowly and deeply, certain physiological changes occur: less oxygen is consumed and less carbon dioxide eliminated; muscle tension is re- duced; and there is a decrease in the activity of the sympathetic nervous system and an increase in para-sympathetic activity. Even a few minutes of deep relaxation will reduce worry and fatigue more effectively than many hours of restless sleep.

The Corpse Pose

The Corpse Pose or Savasana is the classic relaxation pose, practised before each session, between asanas, and in Final Relaxation (p.26). It looks deceptively simple, but it is in fact one of the most difficult asanas to do well and one which changes and develops with practice. At the end of an asana session your Corpse Pose will be more complete than at the beginning because the other asanas will have progressively stretched and relaxed your muscles. When you first lie down, look to see that you are lying symmetrically as symmetry provides proper space for all parts to relax. Now start to work into the pose. Rotate your legs in and out, then let them fall gently out to the sides. Do the same with your arms. Rotate the spine by turning your head from side to side to centre it. Then start stretching yourself out, as though someone were pulling your head away from your feet, your shoulders down and away from your neck, your legs down away from your pelvis. Let gravity embrace you. Feel your weight pulling you deeper into relaxation, melting your body into the floor. Breathe deeply and slowly from the abdomen (right), riding up and down on the breath, sinking deeper with each exhalation. Feel how your abdomen swells and falls. Many important physiological changes are taking place, reducing the body's energy loss, removing stress, lowering your respiration and pulse rate, and resting the whole system. As you enter deep relaxation, you will feel your mind grow clear and detached.

The Corpse Pose (right)
Lie on your back, feet spread about 18 inches apart and hands about 6 inches from your sides, palms up. Ease yourself into the pose, making sure the body is symmetrical. Let your thighs, knees and toes turn outward. Close your eyes and breathe deeply.

Abdominal Breathing
To check that you are breathing correctly, exhale and place your hands on your abdomen, fingers loosely interlocked. When you inhale, your abdomen should rise up, separating your hands.

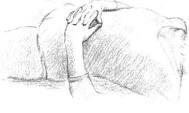

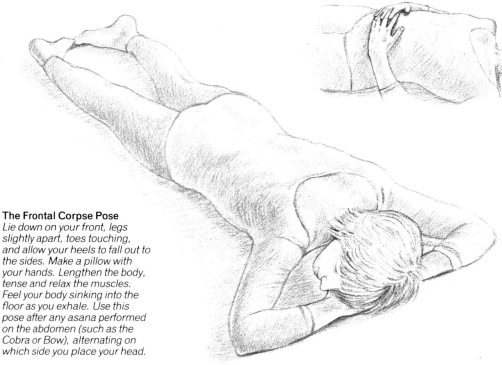

The Frontal Corpse Pose
Lie down on your front, legs slightly apart, toes touching, and allow your heels to fall out to the sides. Make a pillow with your hands. Lengthen the body, tense and relax the muscles. Feel your body sinking into the floor as you exhale. Use this pose after any asana performed on the abdomen (such as the Cobra or Bow), alternating on which side you place your head.

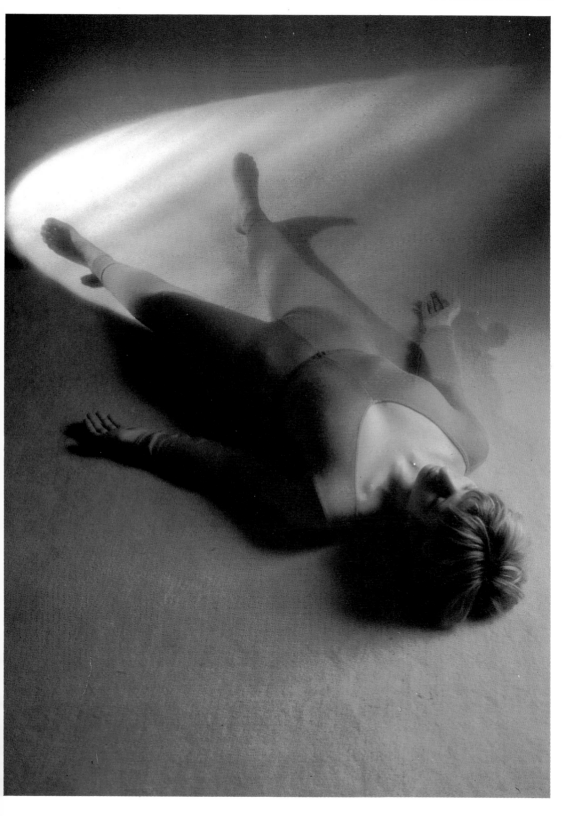

Final Relaxation

Your yoga practice will help you to be more in touch with your body, able to recognize tension and relaxation and thus to bring them under your conscious control. At the end of a session of asanas, you should spend at least ten minutes in Final Relaxation. During this time, you relax each part of the body in turn. But in order to experience relaxation, you must first experience tension. Working up from the feet, as shown below, you first tense and lift each part, then drop (but don't place) it down. Now let your mind travel throughout the body, commanding each part to relax. Let yourself go. Sink deep into the quiet pool of the mind. To bring your consciousness back to your body, gently move your fingers and toes, take a deep breath and as you exhale, sit up.

Hands and arms *Raise your right hand an inch off the floor. Make a fist, tense the arm, then let it drop. Repeat on the other side. Relax.*

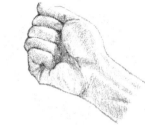

Feet and legs *Lift your right foot just an inch off the floor. Tense the leg, hold, then let it drop. Repeat on the other side.*

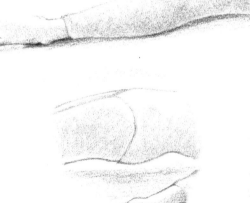

Buttocks *Clench your buttocks tightly together, lift the hips a little way off the floor and hold. Relax and drop them down.*

Chest *Tense and lift up the back and chest, keeping your hips and head on the floor. Relax and drop them down.*

Face *Squeeze every muscle in your face up tight, bringing it to a point around the nose. Now open the face wide, stretching* *your eyes open, and stick out your tongue as far as it will go. Relax.*

Auto-suggestion

After practising the sequence shown, visualize your body in your mind's eye, and repeat this simple formula mentally: "I relax the toes, I relax the toes. The toes *are* relaxed. I relax the calves. I relax the calves. The calves *are* relaxed" Continue on up the body, applying the formula to each part along the way – the stomach, lungs, heart, jaw, scalp, brain, etc. Feel a wave of relaxation rising up your body as you guide your awareness through each part. Each time you inhale feel a wave of oxygen flowing down to your feet; each time you exhale, feel the tension flowing out of your body, leaving your mind like a deep, still lake, without a ripple. Now dive deep in to the centre of this lake, deep within yourself, and experience your true nature.

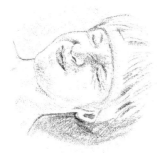

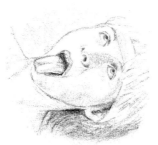

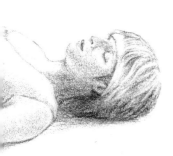

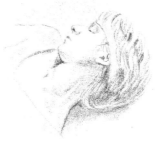

Head *Tuck in your chin slightly and roll the head gently from side to side. Find a comfortable position in the centre for the head to lie, and then relax.*

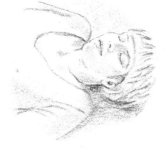

Shoulders *Lift your shoulders and hunch them up tight around your neck. Let them drop, relaxed. Now pull each arm, in turn, down alongside the body, and relax.*

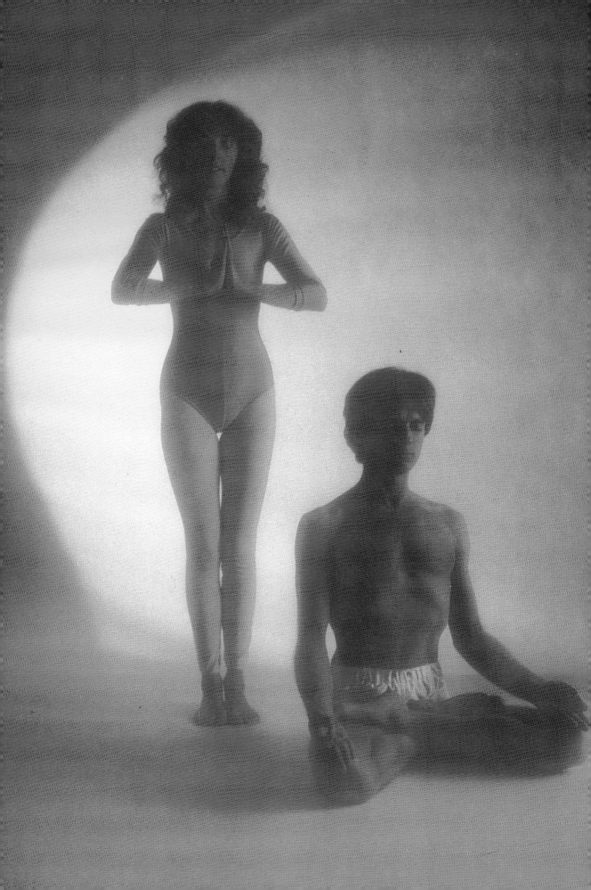

The Basic Session

"Asanas make one firm, free from
maladies, and light of limb."
Hatha Yoga Pradipika

This chapter provides you with the basic set of yoga asanas or postures which form the foundation of your daily practice. To understand the nature of the asanas, you need to experience their effects for yourself. Asanas are postures to be held, rather than exercises, and are performed slowly and meditatively, combined with deep abdominal breathing. These gentle movements not only reawaken your awareness and control of your body, but also have a profound effect spiritually – freeing you from fears and helping to instil confidence and serenity. At the end of a yoga session, you will find yourself relaxed and full of energy – quite unlike after other forms of physical exercise which cause fatigue through overexertion.

There are three stages to each asana – coming into the pose, holding it, and coming out of it. For clarity we have taught you how to come into the pose correctly by showing a number of steps. None of these preliminary steps are meant to be held, unless otherwise stated – you should perform them as one continuous movement into the final position. The real work of an asana is done while you hold the position – adepts of yoga will remain motionless in a pose for hours at a stretch. Try to keep still while you maintain the pose and breathe slowly and deeply, concentrating your mind. Once you are able to relax in a pose, you can adjust your position to achieve a greater stretch. Always release your body from an asana with as much grace and control as you used to come into it.

Asanas work on all the various systems of the body, creating suppleness in the spine and joints and toning the muscles, glands, and internal organs. Though at first it will be the physical experience of the postures that affects you most strongly, as you progress you will grow more and more aware of the flow of prana, the vital energy, and of the importance of correct breathing – pranayama. The ultimate purpose of both asanas and pranayama is to purify the nadis or nerve channels so that prana can flow freely through them, and to prepare the body for the raising of Kundalini, the supreme cosmic energy, which leads the yogi to a state of God consciousness.

The basic session is suitable for all ages and levels of students – from complete beginners to those of you who already have several years' experience. If you are just starting, follow the basic course on pages 66-67 for the first few weeks. Don't be discouraged if your progress seems slow at first and your asanas seem to bear little resemblance to those we have illustrated. Regular practice will steadily narrow the gap. Picture yourself performing an asana perfectly, even if you have not yet mastered it. By approaching each asana positively and using your powers of visualization, you can speed up your progress considerably. Above all, never risk injury by forcing your body into a position or straining to go further than you are presently able. It is only when your muscles are relaxed that they will stretch and allow you to advance in a posture.

Lastly, although we have presented the asanas as clearly as possible, no book can give you the live feedback of a teacher – so try to attend a class whenever you can, to check that you are performing the poses correctly and to learn how to pace your breathing exercises and asanas. You will gain inspiration too, from observing and talking to students who are more advanced than yourself.

The Sequence of Asanas

When you practise Hatha Yoga, it is very important to work according to a pattern. The sequence given here, devised by Swami Vishnu, is a comprehensive series of warm-ups and asanas, based on a strong scientific foundation. It is designed to maintain the proper curvature of the spine, and keep all systems of the body healthy (see pp. 176 – 187). During the sequence the entire body is bent, stretched and toned. Each asana augments or counterbalances the one before. Each series of asanas is followed by one that provides the opposite stretch. Thus, the three backward bends – the Cobra, Locust and Bow – lead on from the Forward Bend. In the same way, any asana that works primarily on one side is always repeated on the other. Whether you are just starting yoga or are already quite advanced, regard the sequence as a pattern on which to build – once you are past the beginning stages you can incorporate new asanas from Asanas and Variations into the sequence (see pp. 100 – 155). Don't worry if you are too short of time to perform all the asanas – the practice chart on page 66 provides a "Half-Hour Class". Now let's look at the elements that make up the sequence.

The session begins with two or three minutes of relaxation in the **Corpse Pose** (see p. 24). You should use this time to relax, breathing deeply and focusing your mind on your breath. Be sure to relax in this pose after every asana until your breathing and heartbeat have returned to normal. (Rest on your abdomen after the Cobra, Locust and Bow.)

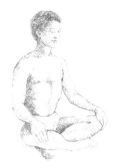

Next you sit up in the **Easy Pose** (or one of the other meditative poses) for pranayama, or the breathing exercises (pp. 68 – 77), which will recharge you with energy. Remaining in the pose, you relieve any stiffness in the upper body by practising **Neck and Shoulder Exercises**, then **Eye Exercises** to strengthen these underused muscles. Now change to a kneeling position for the **Lion Pose**, which releases tension from the neck and throat.

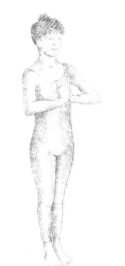

To perform the **Sun Salutation** you rise to your feet. The bending and stretching movements of this sequence of twelve asanas warm up and tone the whole body, bringing flexibility to the spine and making the other asanas in the sequence easier to accomplish.

Now lie down to practise a series of **Leg Raises**. These strengthen the muscles of the abdomen and lower back, and so prepare the body for the Headstand.

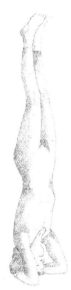

In the **Headstand** – one of the most important asanas – only the head and forearms make contact with the floor and the body is completely inverted. Holding this position brings tremendous benefits.

Next comes a series of three postures – the Shoulderstand, Plough and Bridge – all of them performed from the same neck and shoulder position. In the **Shoulderstand**, the body is once again inverted and the torso and legs raised straight up, as in the Headstand, but now the weight of the body is taken by the shoulders, upper arms, head and neck, and the upper spine and neck are stretched. The **Plough** increases the stretch on the neck

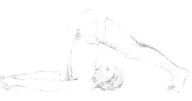

and upper spine and bends the spine forward, bringing the feet to rest behind the head. In the **Bridge**, the torso swings over to bring the feet down in front of the body, arching the spine in the opposite direction to the Plough. As a beginner you will need to relax in the Corpse Pose between these three asanas. But with practice you will gain enough control and flexibility to come down from the Shoulder-stand to the Plough, then go back into the Shoulderstand and straight into the Bridge before it is necessary for you to lie down and relax.

The **Fish** acts as a counterpose to the previous three asanas, compressing instead of stretching the neck and upper spine, and relieving local stiffness.

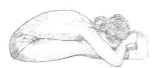

Next comes the **Forward Bend.** This augments the Plough pose, but here it is the base rather than the top of the spine that receives the greatest stretch. This is followed by a series of

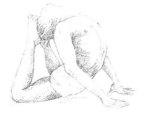

three asanas performed on the abdomen – the Cobra, Locust and Bow, which between them bring flexibility to the whole back. In the **Cobra**, the head

and upper part of the body are raised and arched back. In the **Locust**, the head and chest remain on the floor while the legs and hips are elevated. The **Bow** combines the movements of the other two backward-bending poses, arching both halves of the body at once, resting only on the abdomen.

Having bent the body forward and backward, you now sit up for the **Half Spinal Twist**, which rotates the body to each side in turn, twisting the spine laterally. Still sitting, you come to one of the most renowned meditative poses, the **Lotus**. In this asana,

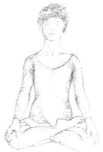

the head, neck and spine remain in a straight line and the legs are locked together to form a steady base, ideal for meditation.

Next comes the **Crow** – a good exercise for balance and for concentration in which only the hands remain on the floor, supporting the whole weight of the body. The asanas end with two standing positions – the **Hands to Feet Pose**, which bends the body forward, inverting the torso; and finally the **Triangle,** which stretches the spine to each side in turn. Every session ends with Final Relaxation. Lying down in the **Corpse Pose** for at least ten

minutes, you relax each part of the body in turn, as described on page 24. It is vital that you integrate this relaxation time into your asana session right from the start. Otherwise the mind may find an excuse to leave it out and you will not absorb the full effects of the asanas.

Practical matters

All you really need to practise asanas is your body and the floor – plus a little self-discipline. Try to get into the habit of doing your asanas at the same time each day – it is more beneficial to do a short sequence daily than a longer session every few days. Set aside a special time that you can devote to yourself, free from distractions of the world outside. Ideal times are in the evening before eating or early in the morning, though you will find your body a little stiffer then. Whatever time you choose, you should always do your asanas on an empty stomach – try not to eat for at least an hour before your session. Practise your asanas on a blanket, wearing comfortable, loose-fitting clothing – tight clothes restrict breathing and circulation. Leave your feet bare and take off your watch and any jewellery. Above all, keep warm as your muscles will stiffen if you get cold. Practise in a well-ventilated room, or, if the weather is suitable, out of doors.

Caution *Women with IUDs should have regular check-ups from their doctors, to ensure that the device has not shifted. Some asanas cause internal movement.*

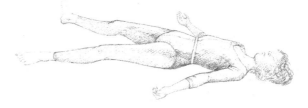

The Session Begins

The Easy Pose

After relaxing in the Corpse Pose for a few minutes, come up and sit in the Easy Pose, Sukhasana, for pranayama (see pp. 68-77) and the neck, shoulder and eye exercises illustrated here. This asana is one of the classic meditative poses which help to straighten the spine, slow the metabolism and still the mind. If you find that holding the pose is uncomfortable, place a folded blanket under the back of your buttocks. In order to stretch the leg muscles evenly, be sure to alternate which leg you place on top in the posture. When you are ready, substitute the Half Lotus or Lotus at this point.

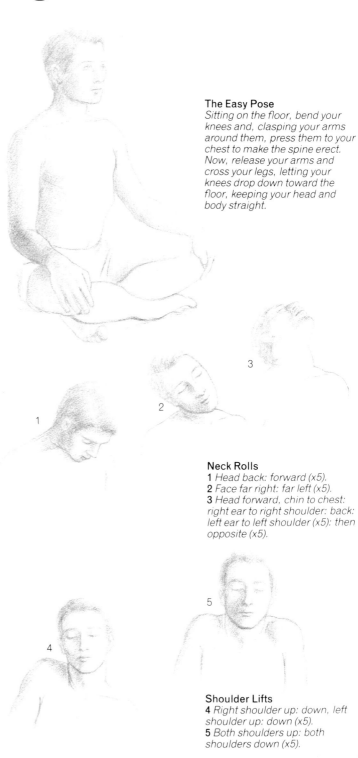

The Easy Pose
Sitting on the floor, bend your knees and, clasping your arms around them, press them to your chest to make the spine erect. Now, release your arms and cross your legs, letting your knees drop down toward the floor, keeping your head and body straight.

3

2

1

Neck Rolls
1 *Head back: forward (x5).*
2 *Face far right: far left (x5).*
3 *Head forward, chin to chest: right ear to right shoulder: back: left ear to left shoulder (x5): then opposite (x5).*

Neck and Shoulders

Many people hold tension in their necks and shoulders, leading to stiffness, bad posture and to tension headaches. Repeating these five exercises eases tension, increases flexibility and tones the muscles. Do them slowly and keep your spine straight, your neck relaxed and your shoulders facing forward. First, drop your head back, then drop it right forward. Now, keeping your head erect, turn it all the way to the right, back to the centre, then all the way to the left. Next, drop your head forward and roll it around in as wide a circle as possible. Repeat in the opposite direction. Now, raise your right shoulder, then drop it down. Repeat with the left. Lastly, raise both shoulders at once, then drop them down again.

5

4

Shoulder Lifts
4 *Right shoulder up: down, left shoulder up: down (x5).*
5 *Both shoulders up: both shoulders down (x5).*

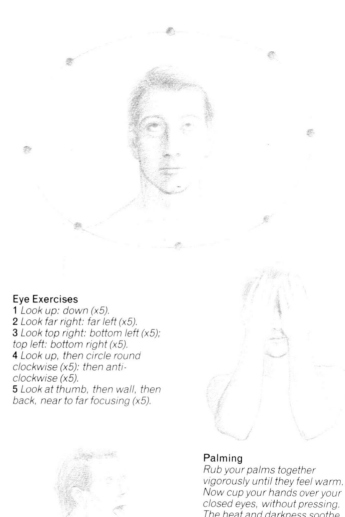

Eye Exercises

Like any other muscles, the eye muscles need exercise if they are to be healthy and strong. Much of the time we only shift our gaze minimally from left to right, as when reading, and turn our heads if we want to look elsewhere. By moving the eyes in every direction, without turning your head at all, these five exercises will strengthen the muscles, and help to prevent eyestrain and improve eyesight. Breathe normally while you are practising them. First, look up, then look down. Now look to the far right, then look far left. Next look up to the right, then look diagonally downward to the left. Repeat in the opposite direction. Now imagine a large clock – look up at 12 o'clock, then circle around it clockwise, quite slowly for two rounds then quicker for three. Repeat the exercise in an anticlockwise direction. Lastly, hold your thumb up about a foot from your face, and move your eyes from the thumb to the wall beyond and back. To end, always "palm" your eyes as shown right.

Eye Exercises
1 *Look up: down (x5).*
2 *Look far right: far left (x5).*
3 *Look top right: bottom left (x5); top left: bottom right (x5).*
4 *Look up, then circle round clockwise (x5): then anti-clockwise (x5).*
5 *Look at thumb, then wall, then back, near to far focusing (x5).*

Palming
Rub your palms together vigorously until they feel warm. Now cup your hands over your closed eyes, without pressing. The heat and darkness soothe and relax your eyes.

The Lion Pose

In Simhasana, the tongue is stretched out to its fullest limit, the eyes rolled upward, and the whole body tensed, like a lion about to spring. Circulation to the tongue and throat is increased, the voice is improved, and the face and throat muscles made stronger. The asana also stimulates the eyes and prepares you for the three bandhas (p. 75). Repeat four to six times.

The Lion Pose
Sit on your heels. Place your hands palms down on your knees, fingers splayed, and inhale through your nose. Now lean slightly forward and exhale forcefully through your mouth, making an AAAH sound. At the same time, stretch your tongue out and down, stretch out your fingers and look up. Hold the pose for as long as you can, then close your mouth and inhale through the nose.

The Sun Salutation

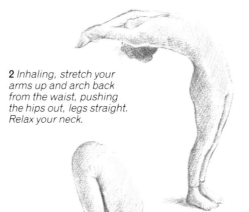

1 *Stand erect with feet together and palms in the prayer position in front of your chest. Make sure your weight is evenly distributed. Exhale.*

The Sun Salutation or Surya Namaskar limbers up the whole body in preparation for the asanas. It is a graceful sequence of twelve positions performed as one continuous exercise. Each position counteracts the one before, stretching the body in a different way and alternately expanding and contracting the chest to regulate the breathing. Practised daily it will bring great flexibility to your spine and joints and trim your waist. One round of Sun Salutation consists of two sequences, the first leading with the right foot in positions 4 and 9, the second leading with the left (as illustrated). Keep your hands in one place from positions 3 to 10 and try to co-ordinate your movements with your breathing. Start by practising four rounds and gradually build up to twelve rounds.

2 *Inhaling, stretch your arms up and arch back from the waist, pushing the hips out, legs straight. Relax your neck.*

3 *Exhaling, fold forward, and press your palms down, fingertips in line with toes – bend your knees if necessary.*

In Hindu mythology, the sun god is worshipped as a symbol of health and immortal life. The Rig Veda declares that "Surya is the Soul, both of the moving and unmoving beings". The Sun Salutation originated as a series of prostrations to the sun. Traditionally, it is performed at dawn, facing the rising sun. In time, each of the twelve positions came to have its own mantra, celebrating aspects of the sun's divinity.

4 *Inhaling, bring the left (or right) leg back and place the knee on the floor. Arch back and look up, lifting your chin.*

5 *Retaining the breath, bring the other leg back and support your weight on hands and toes. Keep your head and body in line and look at the floor between your hands.*

6 *Exhaling, lower your knees, then your chest and then your forehead, keeping your hips up and your toes curled under.*

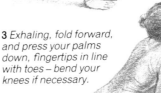

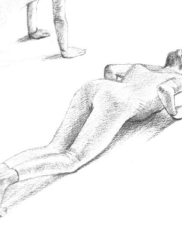

12 *Exhaling, gently come back to an upright position and bring your arms down by your sides.*

11 *Inhaling, stretch your arms forward, then up and back over your head and bend back slowly from the waist, as in position 2.*

10 *Exhaling, bring the other leg forward and bend down from the waist, keeping your palms as in position 3.*

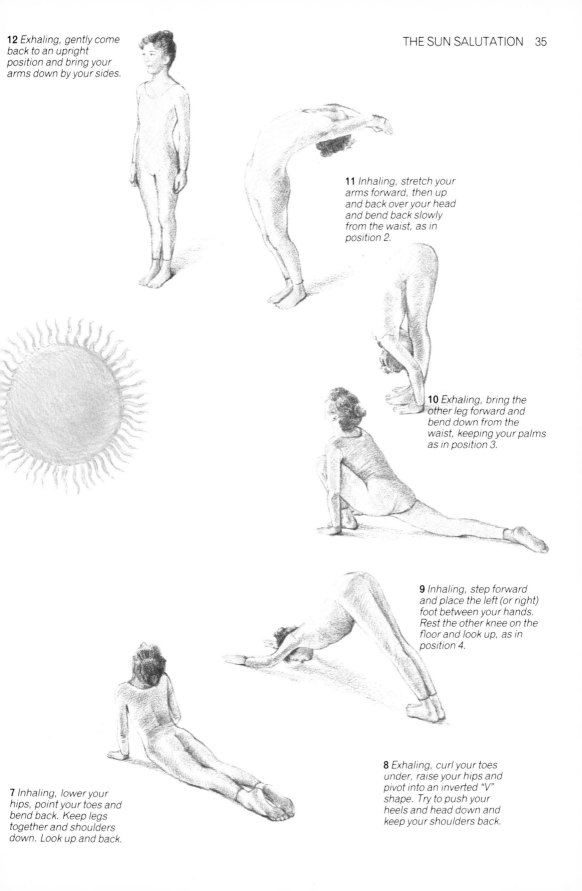

9 *Inhaling, step forward and place the left (or right) foot between your hands. Rest the other knee on the floor and look up, as in position 4.*

8 *Exhaling, curl your toes under, raise your hips and pivot into an inverted "V" shape. Try to push your heels and head down and keep your shoulders back.*

7 *Inhaling, lower your hips, point your toes and bend back. Keep legs together and shoulders down. Look up and back.*

Leg Raises

These simple exercises prepare the body for asanas, strengthening in particular the abdominal and lower back muscles used to come up into the Headstand and trimming the waist and thighs. If your muscles are weak, you may find yourself arching your lower back or using your shoulders to help lift your legs, To get the most benefit from the exercises, make sure that the full length of your back is resting on the floor and keep shoulders and neck relaxed. All of these exercises begin with legs together and palms down by your sides.

Single Leg Raising

In this series, one leg is raised while the other remains flat on the floor. At first you can push down with your hands to help lift your leg. Once your muscles are stronger, leave your hands palms up by your sides. Keep both knees straight and press your lower back down to the floor to straighten the spine.

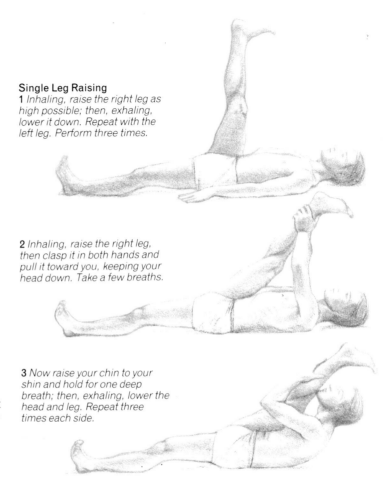

Single Leg Raising
1 Inhaling, raise the right leg as high possible; then, exhaling, lower it down. Repeat with the left leg. Perform three times.

2 Inhaling, raise the right leg, then clasp it in both hands and pull it toward you, keeping your head down. Take a few breaths.

3 Now raise your chin to your shin and hold for one deep breath; then, exhaling, lower the head and leg. Repeat three times each side.

Single Wind Relieving
1 Inhaling, bend the right knee, wrap your hands around it and press to chest. Exhaling, release it. Repeat with the left leg.

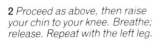

2 Proceed as above, then raise your chin to your knee. Breathe; release. Repeat with the left leg.

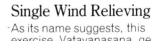

Single Wind Relieving

As its name suggests, this exercise, Vatayanasana, gently massages the digestive system and gives relief from excess wind in the stomach and intestines. It also tones and stretches the lower back. While practising it, resist the tendency to raise the lower back or buttocks off the ground. Try to keep the leg that is on the floor as straight as possible.

Double Leg Raising

This is the most demanding of the leg raises shown here, especially if your abdominal muscles are underdeveloped. At first you may not be able to raise your legs right up or may have to bend your knees slightly while raising the legs, straightening them once they are up. Pressing down with your palms will help you to lift the legs. If you have a particular weakness in your lower back or abdominal muscles, try interlocking your fingers and placing them on your abdomen to create an extra set of "muscles". Press the fingers down each time you need to contract the abdominal muscles. Whichever method you adopt, be sure to keep your lower back and buttocks on the floor. Once you can perform double leg raising without strain, lower your legs as slowly as possible and keep your feet an inch or so off the floor between raises to make your muscles work harder.

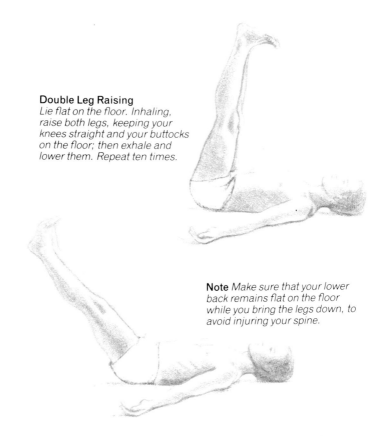

Double Leg Raising
Lie flat on the floor. Inhaling, raise both legs, keeping your knees straight and your buttocks on the floor; then exhale and lower them. Repeat ten times.

Note *Make sure that your lower back remains flat on the floor while you bring the legs down, to avoid injuring your spine.*

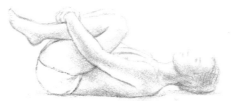

Double Wind Relieving
1 *Inhaling, bend your knees, wrap your hands around them and press them to your chest. Exhaling, release the legs.*

2 *Inhaling, bring your knees in to your chest, as before, then raise the chin to the knees. Now rock gently backward and forward and from side to side. Exhaling, release the legs.*

Double Wind Relieving

Like the single leg version, opposite, this exercise also massages the abdominal organs and helps to release any gases from the intestines. In position 1 keep your head and shoulders down and push your lower back against the floor. When you perform the rocking movement, try to maintain a steady and controlled rhythm. Rocking gets rid of any stiffness in the spine by gently massaging the spinal vertebrae, back muscles and surrounding ligaments.

The Headstand

King of asanas, the Headstand or Sirshasana is one of the most powerfully beneficial postures for both body and mind. By reversing the normal effects of gravity, it rests the heart, aids your circulation, and relieves pressure on the lower back. Practised regularly, it will help prevent back problems and improve memory, concentration, and the sensory faculties. Inverting the body also makes you breathe deeply, bringing a fresh supply of oxygen-rich blood to the brain – any slight breathing difficulty you experience at first will quickly pass. Mastering the Headstand requires no great strength. It is largely a matter of conquering your fears and believing you can do it. The key to balance is the tripod formed by elbows and hands – make sure your elbows don't shift out of position.

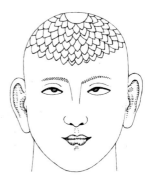

"He who practises the Headstand for three hours daily conquers time."
Yoga Tattva Upanishad

1 Kneel down and rest your weight on your forearms. Wrap your hands around your elbows.
2 Release your hands and place them in front of you, with fingers interlocked. Your elbows now stay in this position.
3 Place the back of your head in your clasped hands and the top of your head on the floor. The hands and elbows form a tripod, making a firm foundation for the inverted body.
4 Now straighten your knees and raise your hips.

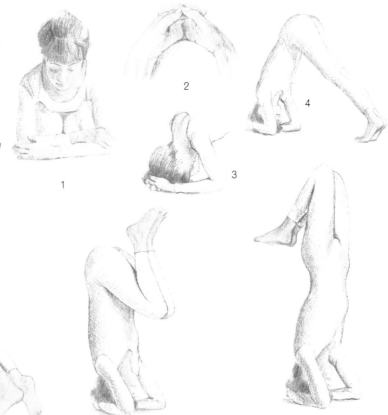

5 Without bending the knees, walk your feet in as close to your head as possible. Pull your hips back so that your neck is not bent backward or forward, but is in a straight line with the spine.

6 Bend your knees in to your chest and lift your feet off the floor, pulling your hips backward as you do so. Pause at this point – do not immediately attempt to raise your knees higher.

7 Then, keeping your knees bent, lift them up toward the ceiling, using your abdominal muscles.

Caution *People with high blood pressure, glaucoma, or a detached retina should concentrate on asanas which may rectify the condition before approaching the Headstand.*

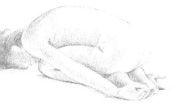

The Child's Pose

This relaxation pose is used to normalise the circulation after the Headstand and to give a counterstretch to the spine after the backward bends. Kneel down and sit back on your feet, heels pointing outward. Place your forehead on the floor, then bring your arms alongside your body, palms turned upward.

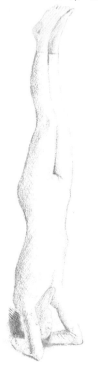

8 *Now slowly straighten your legs. You will feel most of the body's weight on the forearms. To come down, reverse steps 5, 6, and 7. Rest in the Child's Pose for at least six deep breaths.*

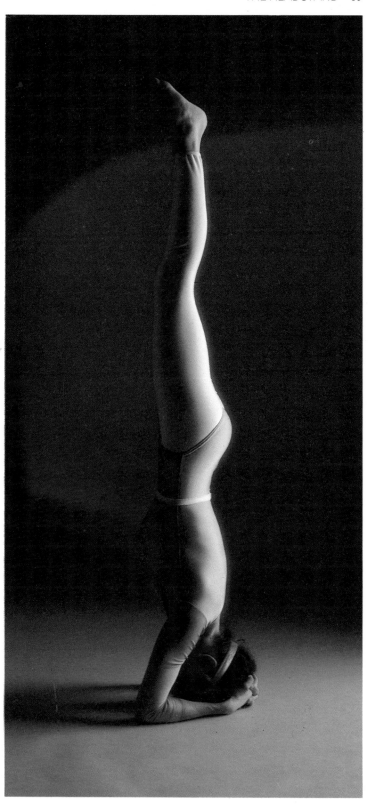

The Shoulderstand

According to Swami Sivananda, three asanas alone will keep the body in perfect health – the Headstand, the Shoulderstand and the Forward Bend. The Shoulderstand invigorates and rejuvenates your whole body – the Sanskrit name Sarvang-asana means literally "all parts pose". An ideal pick-me-up, it gives many of the same benefits as the Headstand, with the difference that inverting the body at right angles to the head stretches the neck and upper spine and, most important, stimulates the thyroid and parathyroid glands by pressing your chin into the base of your throat. The pose encourages deep abdominal breathing because it limits use of the top of your lungs. Initially this may feel a little constricting, but you will soon adapt as you relax into the pose. To come out of the Shoulderstand, always use the roll-out described below.

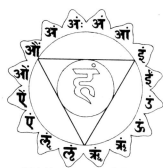

"This Yoga must be followed with faith, with a strong and courageous heart."
Bhagavad Gita

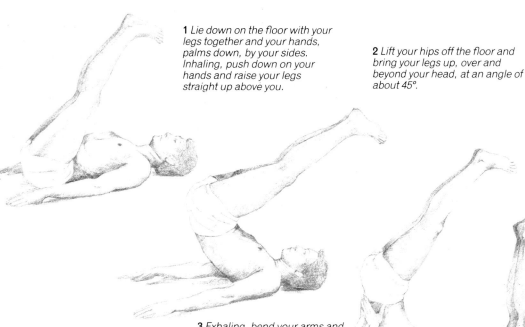

1 *Lie down on the floor with your legs together and your hands, palms down, by your sides. Inhaling, push down on your hands and raise your legs straight up above you.*

2 *Lift your hips off the floor and bring your legs up, over and beyond your head, at an angle of about 45°.*

3 *Exhaling, bend your arms and support your body, holding as near the shoulders as possible, thumbs around the front of the body, fingers around the back. Push your back up, lift your legs.*

Shoulderstand roll-out

To come down from the pose, lower your legs to an angle of about 45° over your head, place your hands palms down behind you, then slowly roll out of it, vertebra by vertebra. Breathe normally until your whole spine is resting on the floor and your legs are at right angles to it, then exhale as you slowly lower your legs, keeping the knees straight.

4 *Now straighten your spine and bring the legs up to a vertical position. Press your chin firmly into the base of your throat. Breathe slowly and deeply in the pose, gradually trying to work your elbows closer together and your hands further down your back toward the shoulders, so as to straighten your torso. Keep your feet relaxed.*

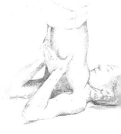

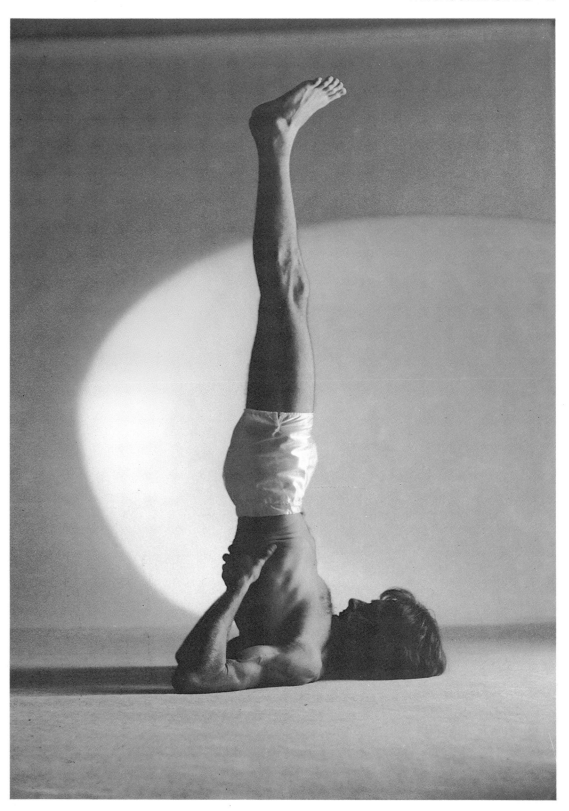

The Plough

The Plough or Halasana completes the movement of the Shoulderstand, bringing the feet and hands down to the floor to mould the body into the shape of a primitive plough. The pose shares many of the Shoulderstand's effects: it gives flexibility to the spine and neck, nourishes the spinal nerves, and strengthens the back, shoulder, and arm muscles while releasing tension. By compressing the abdomen, it also massages the internal organs. When you perform the Plough, be sure to keep your spine stretched up and your knees straight. Your feet may not reach the floor to begin with, but as your spine becomes more supple, the weight of your legs will gradually pull them down. Advanced students can go straight into the pose from the Shoulderstand, but beginners should relax in between. Use the Shoulderstand roll-out to come out of the Plough.

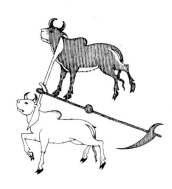

"Sow love, reap peace: . . . Sow meditation, reap wisdom."
Swami Sivananda

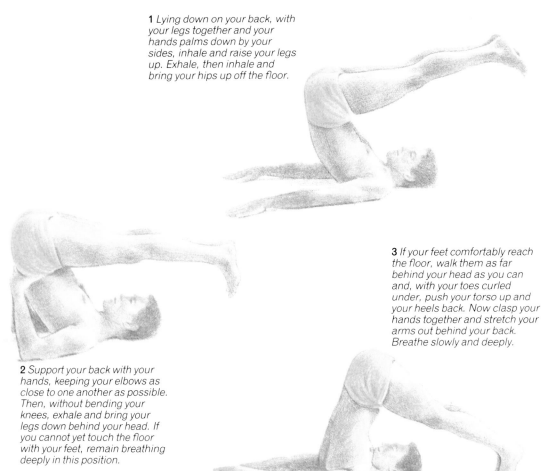

1 *Lying down on your back, with your legs together and your hands palms down by your sides, inhale and raise your legs up. Exhale, then inhale and bring your hips up off the floor.*

3 *If your feet comfortably reach the floor, walk them as far behind your head as you can and, with your toes curled under, push your torso up and your heels back. Now clasp your hands together and stretch your arms out behind your back. Breathe slowly and deeply.*

2 *Support your back with your hands, keeping your elbows as close to one another as possible. Then, without bending your knees, exhale and bring your legs down behind your head. If you cannot yet touch the floor with your feet, remain breathing deeply in this position.*

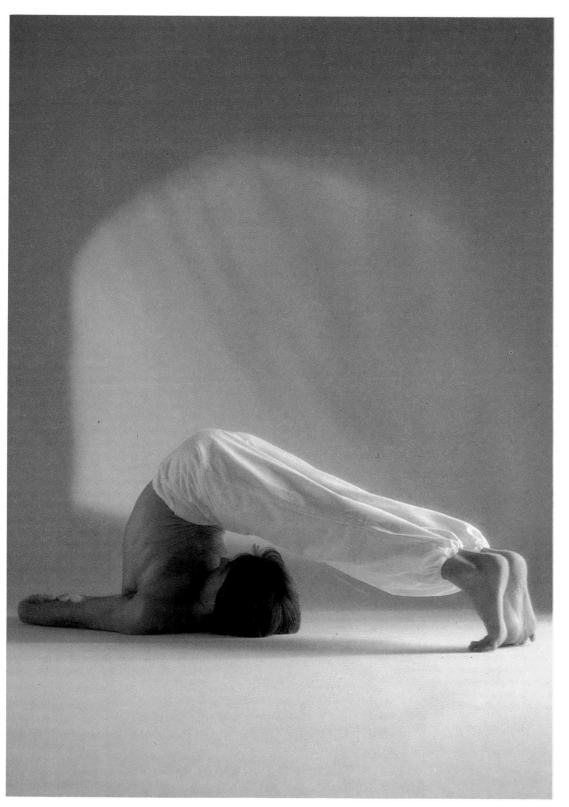

The Bridge

Complementing the Plough, the Bridge brings the feet down from the Shoulderstand in the opposite direction, reversing the stretch on the spine and relieving pressure on the neck. Its Sanskrit name, Sethu Bandhasana, means "bridge-building pose", referring to the way the body creates a perfect arch from head to toe. Moving into and out of the pose strengthens the abdominal and lower back muscles and makes the spine and wrists more supple. To come into the Bridge from the Shoulderstand you need a fairly flexible back – at first you may have to push up into the pose from the floor, as shown below right. Advanced students can perform the Shoulderstand, Plough and Bridge as one continuous series.

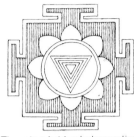

"There is a bridge between time and eternity; and this bridge is Atman, the Spirit of man."
Chandogya Upanishad

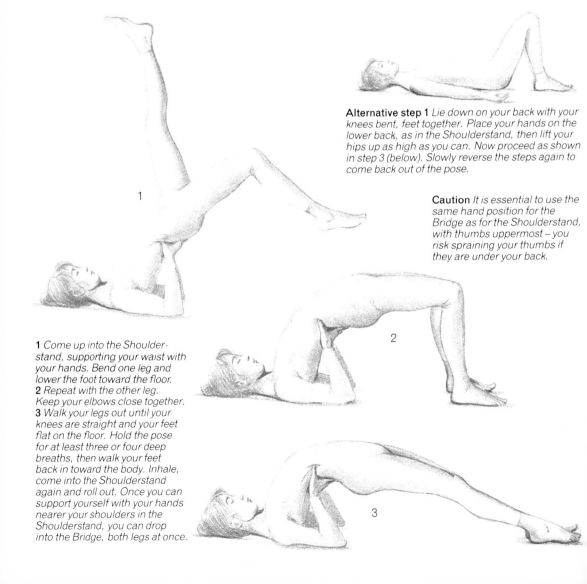

Alternative step 1 *Lie down on your back with your knees bent, feet together. Place your hands on the lower back, as in the Shoulderstand, then lift your hips up as high as you can. Now proceed as shown in step 3 (below). Slowly reverse the steps again to come back out of the pose.*

Caution *It is essential to use the same hand position for the Bridge as for the Shoulderstand, with thumbs uppermost – you risk spraining your thumbs if they are under your back.*

1

2

3

1 *Come up into the Shoulderstand, supporting your waist with your hands. Bend one leg and lower the foot toward the floor.*
2 *Repeat with the other leg. Keep your elbows close together.*
3 *Walk your legs out until your knees are straight and your feet flat on the floor. Hold the pose for at least three or four deep breaths, then walk your feet back in toward the body. Inhale, come into the Shoulderstand again and roll out. Once you can support yourself with your hands nearer your shoulders in the Shoulderstand, you can drop into the Bridge, both legs at once.*

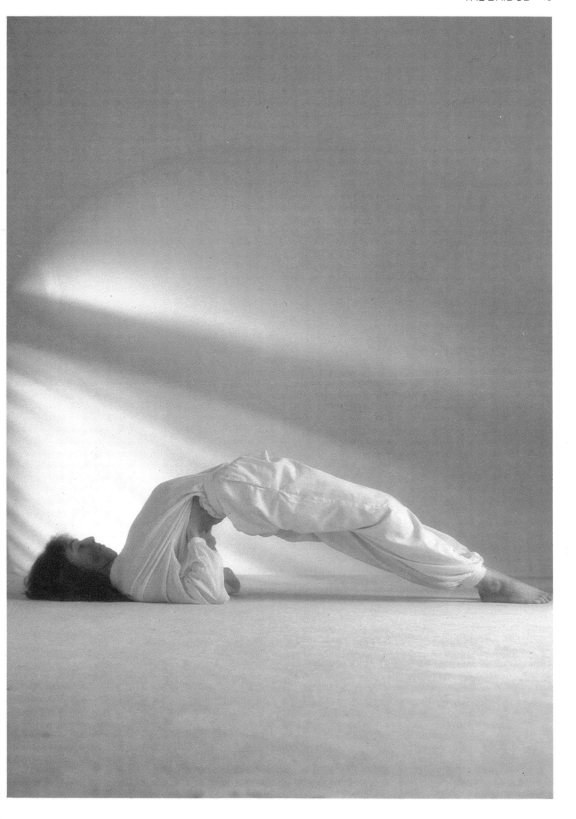

The Fish

Matsya, the fish, was one of the incarnations of the Hindu god Vishnu who assumed this form to save the world from the Flood. The Fish pose, Matsyasana, is the counterpose to the Shoulderstand and must always be practised after it. Having stretched the neck and upper spine in the Shoulderstand, Plough and Bridge, you now compress them as you arch back, relieving stiffness in your neck and shoulder muscles and correcting any tendency to rounded shoulders. Holding the pose exercises the chest, tones the nerves of the neck and back, and ensures that the thyroid and parathyroid glands obtain maximum benefit from the Shoulderstand. It also expands the ribcage fully and so aids deep breathing and increases your lung capacity. You should remain in the pose for at least half the amount of time that you spent in the Shoulderstand in order to balance the stretch.

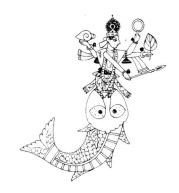

"He who swims across the ocean of time sees the grace of the Lord."
Swami Vishnu Devananda

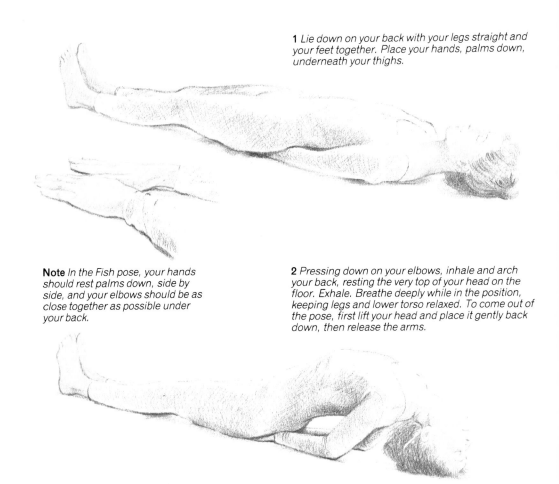

1 *Lie down on your back with your legs straight and your feet together. Place your hands, palms down, underneath your thighs.*

Note *In the Fish pose, your hands should rest palms down, side by side, and your elbows should be as close together as possible under your back.*

2 *Pressing down on your elbows, inhale and arch your back, resting the very top of your head on the floor. Exhale. Breathe deeply while in the position, keeping legs and lower torso relaxed. To come out of the pose, first lift your head and place it gently back down, then release the arms.*

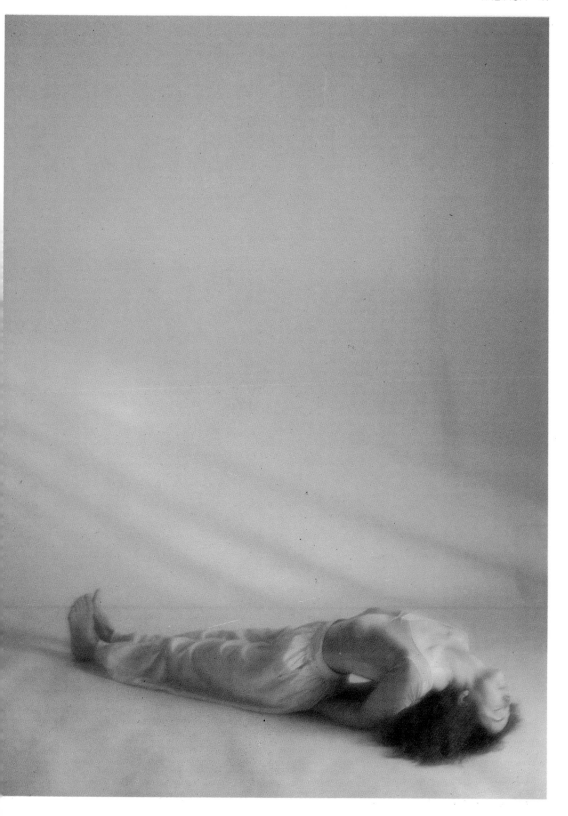

The Forward Bend

The Forward Bend or Paschimothanasana looks deceptively simple. But it is in fact a very important and demanding pose. The Sanskrit word "paschima" means "the West", referring to the back of the body, which is literally stretched from the heels to the top of the spine. Practising this asana invigorates the internal organs, reduces fat, and stimulates the entire nervous system. Before holding the pose, loosen the body up by inhaling and coming back out of the position, then exhaling and going into it again, three times. Don't try to bring your head to your knees as this will curve the spine. Instead, aim to bring the torso as far forward as possible, while keeping knees and spine straight.

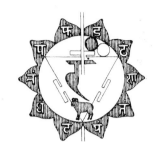

"This most excellent of all asanas . . . makes the breath flow through the Sushumna, stimulates the gastric fire, makes the loins lean and removes all the diseases of men."
Hatha Yoga Pradipika

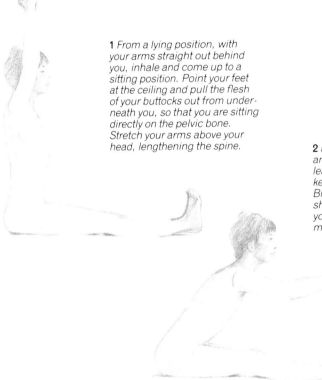

1 *From a lying position, with your arms straight out behind you, inhale and come up to a sitting position. Point your feet at the ceiling and pull the flesh of your buttocks out from underneath you, so that you are sitting directly on the pelvic bone. Stretch your arms above your head, lengthening the spine.*

2 *Pulling the abdomen in, exhale and fold forward from the pelvis, leading with the chest and keeping your back straight. Bring your chin toward your shins and your chest toward your thighs. Don't bend from the middle of your spine.*

3 *Continue right down and hold on to whichever part of your legs or feet you can comfortably reach without bending the knees. With practice, you can wrap your index fingers around your big toes and bring your elbows down to the floor, or stretch your arms out over your feet, as shown right.*

In the position, *breathe deeply, feeling yourself advancing forward a little more every time you exhale. Hold for three to four deep breaths at first, gradually increasing the number as you become relaxed in the pose. When you release the position, reach forward as you come up.*

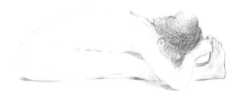

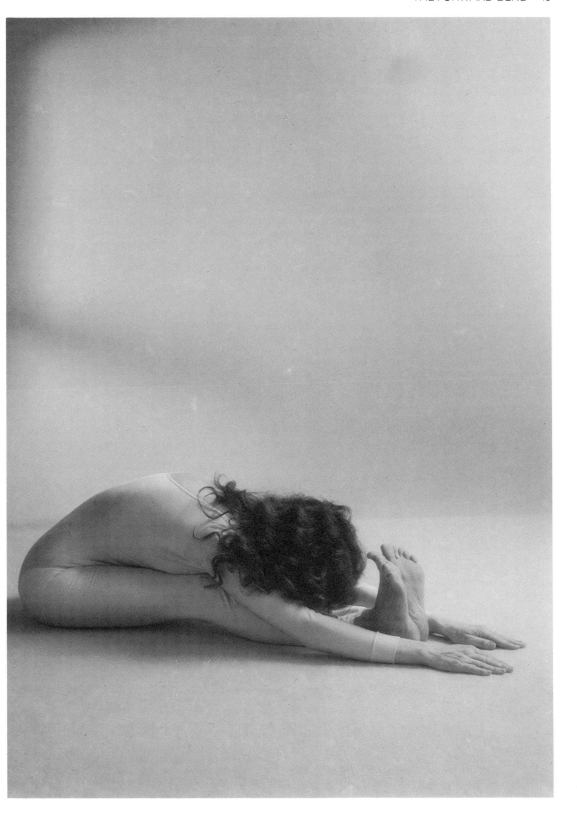

The Cobra

In Bhujangasana, the head and trunk arch gracefully up, like a cobra with its hood raised. The spine receives a powerful backward stretch, the surrounding musculature is strengthened and the abdominal organs are toned up and massaged. The pose is particularly effective for combating menstrual irregularities and pain and relieving constipation. Perform the asana in stages, as shown below, visualizing the smooth, supple movement of a snake as you slowly stretch your spine up and backward, vertebra by vertebra. Keep your shoulders down, your elbows tucked in to your body, and your face relaxed in the pose. You may find the full Cobra position difficult to achieve at first, but in time your spine will become supple enough for head and feet to touch.

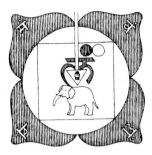

"By the practice of this posture the serpent-goddess (the Kundalini force) awakes."
Gheranda Samhita

1 *Lie down with your legs together and your hands palms down under your shoulders. Rest your forehead on the floor.*
2 *Inhaling, bring your head up, brushing first your nose, then your chin against the floor. Now lift up your hands and use your back muscles to raise your chest as high as possible. Hold for a few deep breaths then, exhaling, slowly return to position 1, keeping your chin up until last.*
3 *Inhaling, come up as before, but this time use your hands to push the trunk up. Continue up until you are bending from the middle of the spine. Hold for two or three deep breaths, then exhale and come slowly down.*

4 *Inhaling, raise the trunk as before, but this time continue up and back until you can feel your back bending all the way down from the neck to the base of the spine. Breathe normally.*

5 *To complete the asana, walk your hands in toward your body, straighten the arms, and lift the pelvis slightly. Separate the legs, bend the knees and, pushing out the chest, drop the head back and touch the feet to the head. Breathe normally, then slowly come down, as before.*

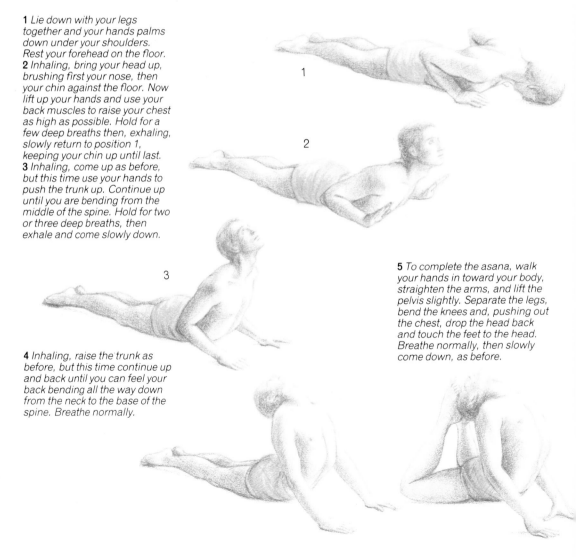

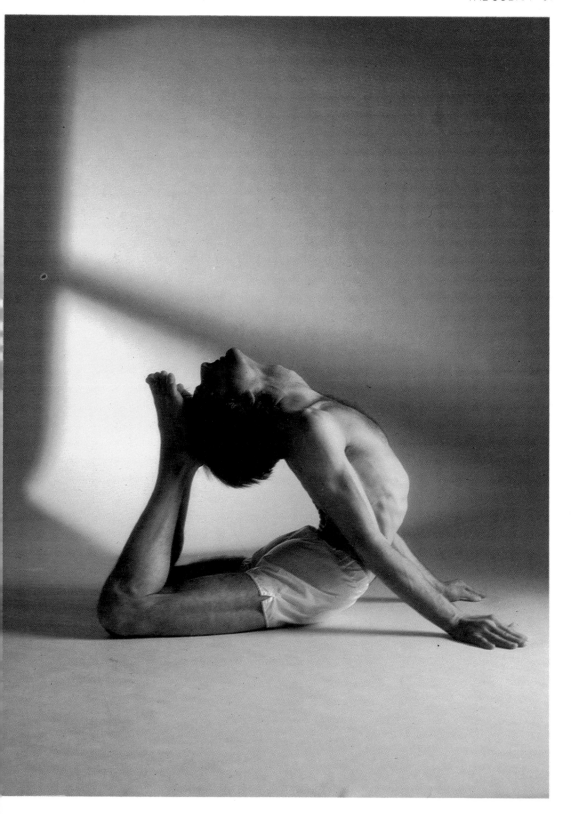

The Locust

Unlike most asanas, the Locust or Salabhasana requires a sudden movement to get into the pose. Its effects supplement those of the Cobra – but where the Cobra concentrates on the upper half of the body, the Locust works mainly on the lower half, strengthening the abdomen, lower back and legs. Like the other backward bends, it massages the internal organs, ensuring efficient functioning of the digestive system and preventing constipation. To begin with, you may only manage to raise your legs a few inches off the floor – in fact, it is at this stage that the pose most resembles a locust, tail in air. With regular practice you will discover how to contract your lower back muscles to thrust your legs up high, as well as developing the necessary strength. In time your legs will come to extend beyond your head, as in the photograph.

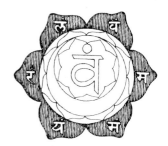

"Truly a flexible back makes for a long life."
Chinese proverb

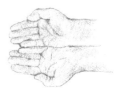

Note *You may find that a different hand position gives you more leverage – with your hands cupped, the palms facing the thighs, as above, or with hands clasped together.*

1 *Lying on your front, inhale and roll on to your side. Make two fists and place them side by side, with thumbs pressing into your thighs. Bring your elbows as close together as possible.*

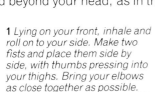

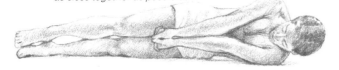

4 *Now take three deep breaths and on the third inhalation, retain the breath and thrust both legs up. Hold the pose, breathing normally, then exhale and bring the legs down with control. Repeat when your breathing has slowed down. Bend your legs, once you can lift them right up. With practice, your feet will rest on your head.*

2 *Exhaling, roll over on to your front, so that you are lying on your arms, with your head resting on your chin. Take a few normal breaths in this position.*

3 *Inhale and raise your right leg, using your hands as a lever. Take two full breaths, then exhale and bring the leg down. Repeat with the left leg. Keep both legs straight and don't swivel the hips.*

Locust

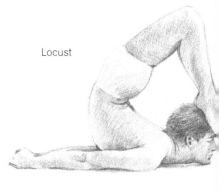

Half Locust

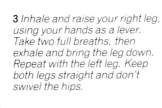

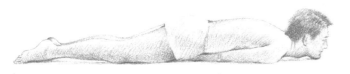

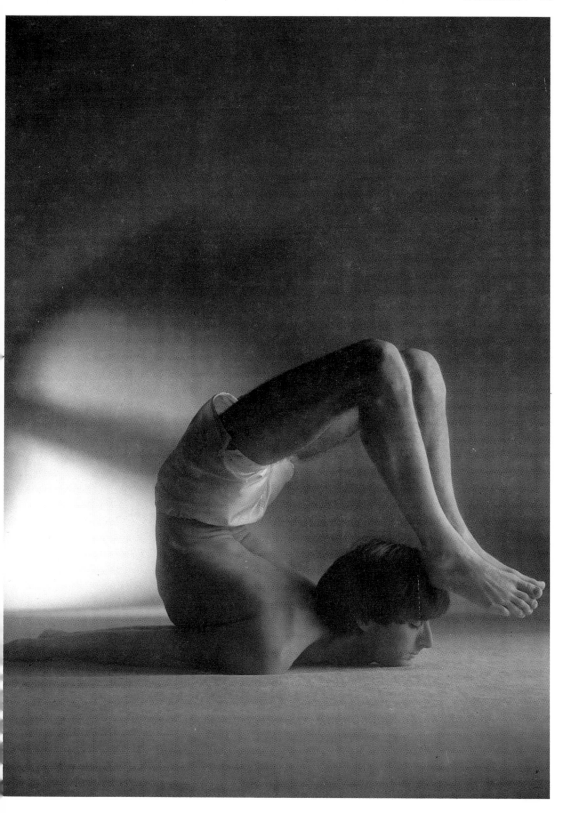

The Bow

The Bow or Dhanurasana raises both halves of the body at once, combining the movements of the Cobra and Locust, and countering the Plough and the Forward Bend. Like an archer stringing a bow, you use your hands and arms to pull your trunk and legs up together to form a curve. This tones your back muscles and maintains the elasticity of your spine, improving posture and increasing vitality. Balancing the weight of the body on your abdomen also reduces abdominal fat and keeps the digestive and reproductive systems healthy. The Rocking Bow, in particular, gives your internal organs a powerful massage. Initially, you will find it easier to lift your knees with legs apart; more advanced students should aim to perform the Bow with legs together.

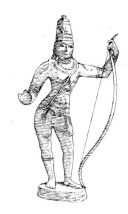

"OM is a bow, the arrow is the Soul,
Brahman is the arrow's goal."
Swami Vishnu Devananda

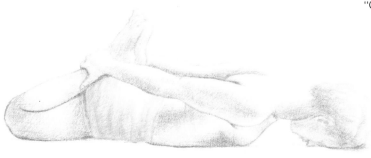

1 *Lie down on your front, head down. Inhale and bend your knees up, then reach back with your hands and clasp hold of your ankles. Exhale.*

2 *Inhaling, raise your head and chest and, simultaneously, pull your ankles up, lifting the knees and thighs off the floor. Arch backward and look up. Take three deep breaths in this pose, then exhale and release it.*

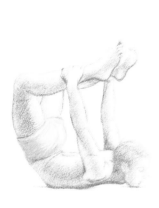

The Rocking Bow
Come into the Bow, then rock forward as you exhale, backward as you inhale. (Don't use your head to rock.) Repeat up to ten times, then relax in the Child's Pose (p.39) for at least six deep breaths.

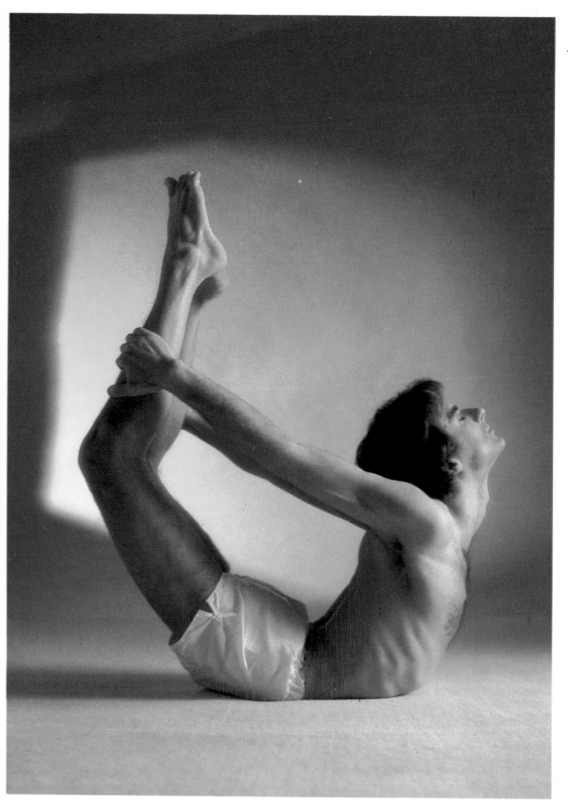

The Half Spinal Twist

The Spinal Twist, which takes its Sanskrit name from the great Yogic sage Matsyendra, is one of the few poses in the Basic Session that rotate the spine. Most bend the spinal column either backward or forward, but to become truly flexible it must be twisted laterally as well. The movement also tones the spinal nerves and ligaments, and improves the digestion. The Half Spinal Twist or Ardha Matsyendrasana, taught here, has similar benefits, and prepares the body for the full pose (p.134). Keep your spine erect and your shoulders level in the position and breathe steadily, twisting a little more each time you exhale. Twist first to the left, as below, then repeat the sequence twisting to the right.

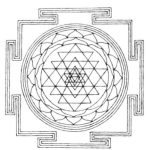

"He who hears the music of
the Soul plays his part
well in life."
Swami Sivananda

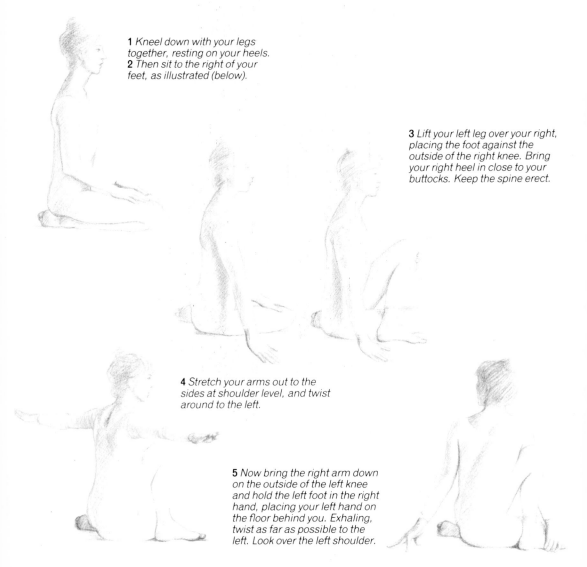

1 *Kneel down with your legs together, resting on your heels.*
2 *Then sit to the right of your feet, as illustrated (below).*

3 *Lift your left leg over your right, placing the foot against the outside of the right knee. Bring your right heel in close to your buttocks. Keep the spine erect.*

4 *Stretch your arms out to the sides at shoulder level, and twist around to the left.*

5 *Now bring the right arm down on the outside of the left knee and hold the left foot in the right hand, placing your left hand on the floor behind you. Exhaling, twist as far as possible to the left. Look over the left shoulder.*

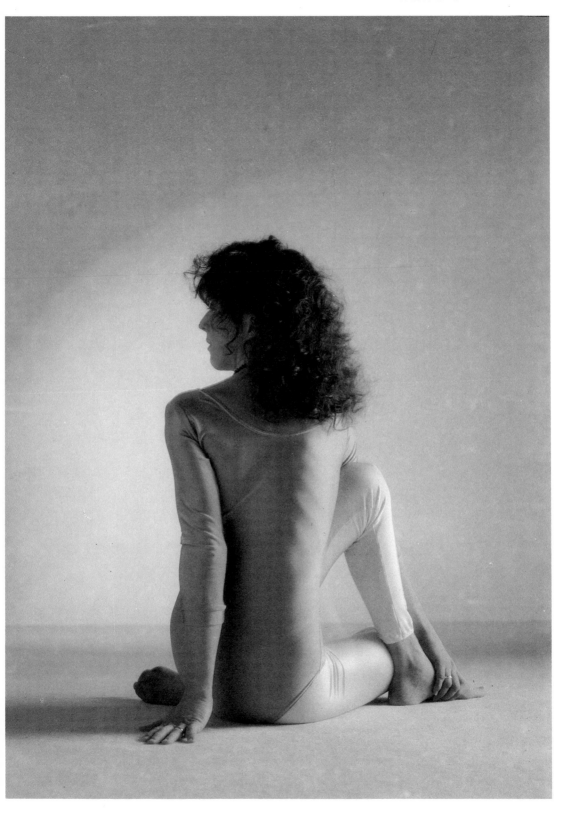

The Lotus

The lotus symbolizes man's spiritual evolution – the roots in mud represent his lower nature, the stem rising through water his intuitive search, and the flower blossoming in sunlight self-realization. In yoga, the Lotus or Padmasana is the classic posture for meditation and pranayama. Sitting with spine erect and legs folded into a steady base brings the body into an effortless, resting state. The longer you hold it, the more the metabolism slows and the mind clears and grows calm. With a straight spine, prana flows smoothly, increasing your powers of concentration. The posture makes ankles, knees and hips more flexible, and benefits the nerves of the legs. Do the Lotus warm-ups and the Half Lotus first.

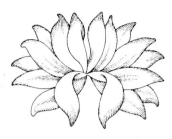

"The yogin seated in the Padmasana posture, by steadying the breath . . . becomes liberated. There is no doubt about this."
Hatha Yoga Pradipika

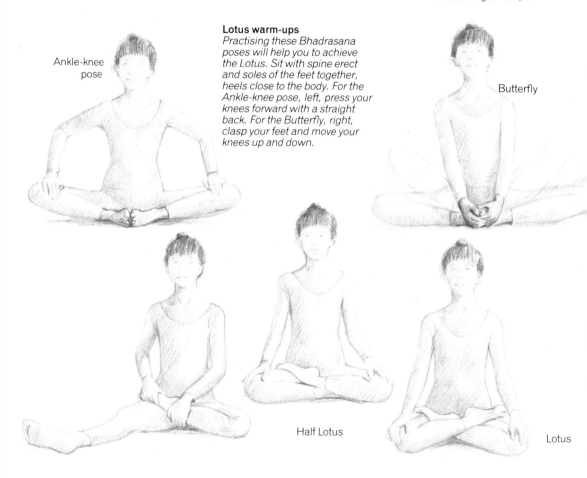

Ankle-knee pose

Lotus warm-ups
Practising these Bhadrasana poses will help you to achieve the Lotus. Sit with spine erect and soles of the feet together, heels close to the body. For the Ankle-knee pose, left, press your knees forward with a straight back. For the Butterfly, right, clasp your feet and move your knees up and down.

Butterfly

Half Lotus

Lotus

The Lotus
To assume the Lotus position, start by sitting with your legs out in a "V" shape in front of you, with spine erect. Bend one knee and bring the foot in, placing it high on the other thigh. Now bring the second foot in. If you place it under the opposite thigh, you form

the Half Lotus (Ardha Padmasana) which is easier at first, and can be used for meditation and pranayama until your legs are more supple. For the full Lotus, you lift the second leg in over the first, placing the foot high on the opposite thigh. In the classic Lotus, the left leg is on top, and the knees touch the floor.

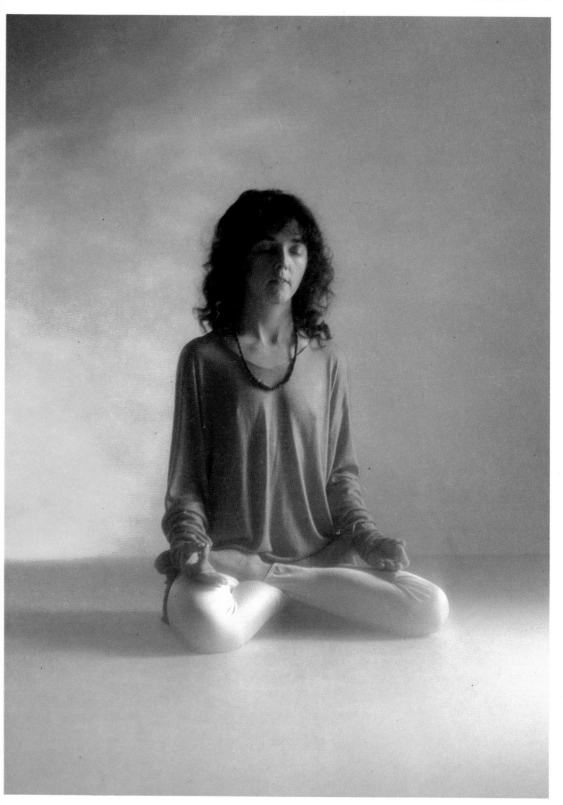

The Crow

This asana strikingly mimics the posture of a cawing crow –
with the body's weight supported on the elbows and hands
and the head thrust well forward. One of the most valuable
balancing poses, the Crow or Kakasana is in fact relatively
easy to achieve, though it may look advanced. The secret is to
lean far enough forward and to keep your mind from
wandering, focusing your attention solely on keeping your
balance. Practising the Crow will greatly strengthen your
wrists, arms, and shoulders, improve your concentration, and
increase your breathing capacity by expanding the chest. (You
will find a wide range of balancing poses in Asanas and
Variations, pp. 100-155.)

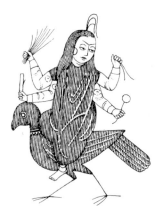

"[The Yogi] sees himself in the heart
of all beings, and all beings in his
heart."
Bhagavad Gita

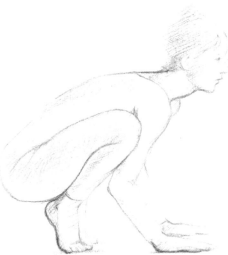

1 *Squat down and bring your
arms between your knees. Place
your palms down flat on the floor
in front of you, shoulder-width
apart, with fingers splayed and
pointing slightly outward. Then
bend your elbows out to the
sides, making the backs of your
arms into shelves for your knees
to rest on.*

2 *Choose a point on the floor in
front of you on which to focus.
Inhale, then while you retain the
breath, lean toward this point,
transferring your weight to your
hands and lifting your toes up.
Exhale and hold the pose for
three or four deep breaths.*

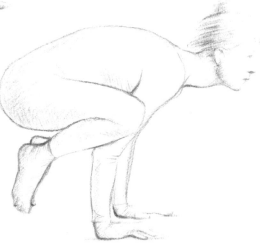

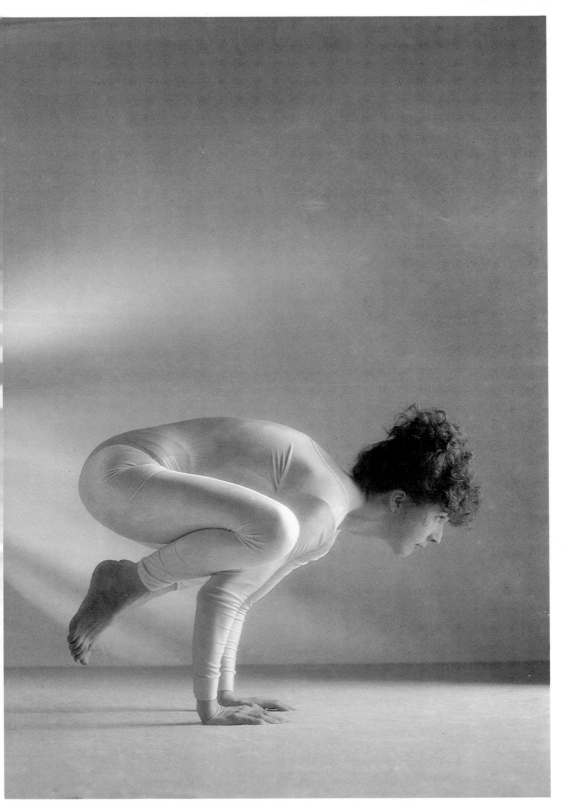

The Hands to Feet Pose

The Hands to Feet Pose or Pada Hastasana gives many of the same benefits as the Forward Bend – trimming the waist, restoring elasticity to the spine, and stretching the ligaments of the legs, especially the hamstrings. It also aids the flow of blood to the brain. Once again, as in the Forward Bend, the purpose of the asana is to bend down as far as you can with your spine and legs straight. Holding your toes and bringing your head in to the shins will follow naturally when your back has become more flexible. Breathe deeply in the position, and let yourself fold a little further down with each exhalation. To pull your chest in closer to your legs, walk your hands back behind you, palms on the floor, as in the photograph.

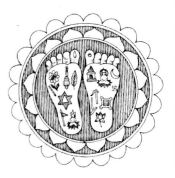

"Nature moulds you constantly into the image of God."
Swami Sivananda

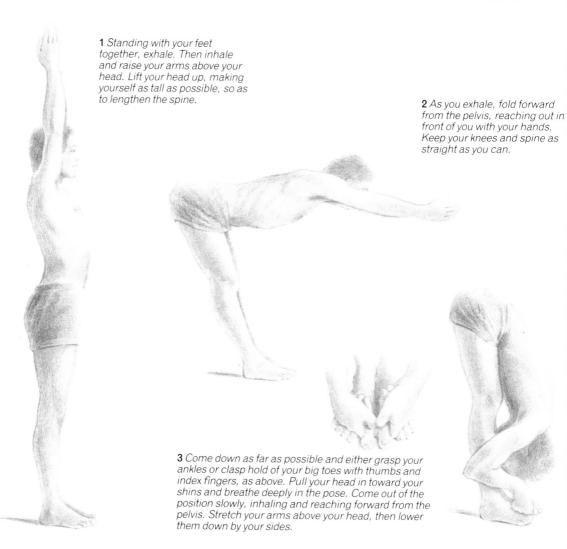

1 *Standing with your feet together, exhale. Then inhale and raise your arms above your head. Lift your head up, making yourself as tall as possible, so as to lengthen the spine.*

2 *As you exhale, fold forward from the pelvis, reaching out in front of you with your hands. Keep your knees and spine as straight as you can.*

3 *Come down as far as possible and either grasp your ankles or clasp hold of your big toes with thumbs and index fingers, as above. Pull your head in toward your shins and breathe deeply in the pose. Come out of the position slowly, inhaling and reaching forward from the pelvis. Stretch your arms above your head, then lower them down by your sides.*

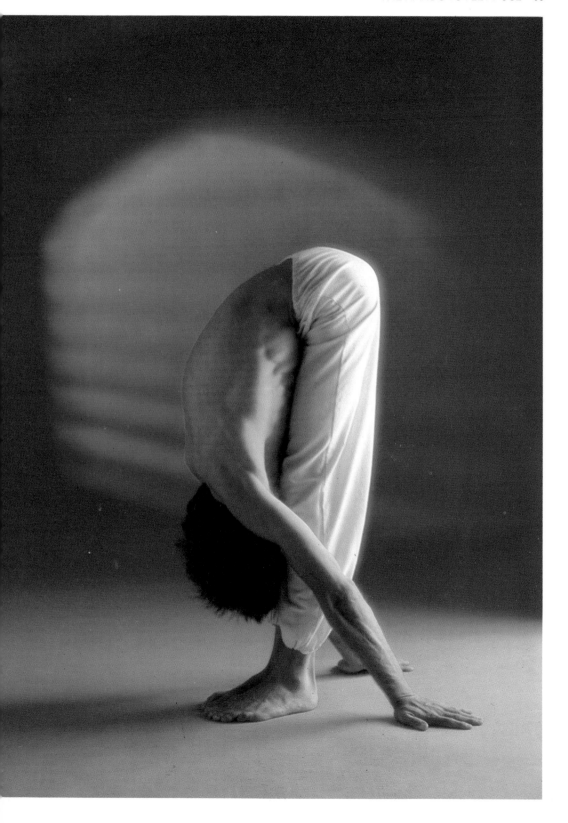

The Triangle

In Hindu art the triangle is a potent symbol for the divine principle, and it is frequently found in the yantras and mandalas used for meditation. Pointing downward it represents Shakti, the dynamic female principle; pointing up it stands for Siva, the passive male force. Trikonasana, the Triangle, concludes the postures in our Basic Session. It augments the movement of the Half Spinal Twist and gives an excellent lateral stretch to the spine, toning the spinal nerves and helping the proper functioning of the digestive system. The body becomes lighter and other asanas are improved. When performing the Triangle, take care that both your knees are straight and that your hips are facing squarely forward, rather than twisted. Bend first to the right, then repeat, bending to the left as shown below. Aim for perfect balance in these basic poses, and you will gain the control and concentration necessary to more advanced variations.

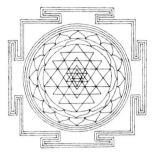

"Joy is eternal, it will never die: sorrow is illusory, it will never live."
Swami Sivananda

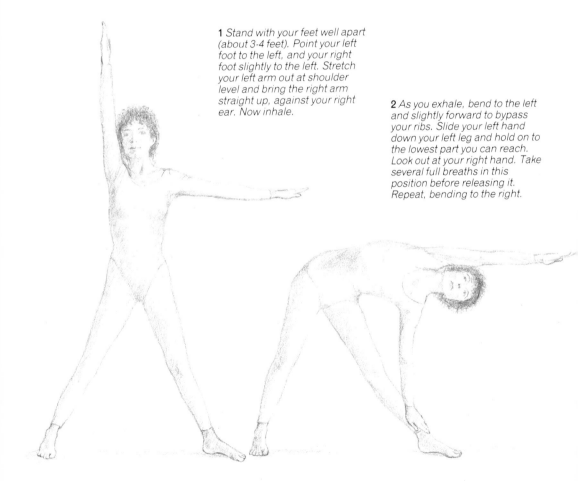

1 *Stand with your feet well apart (about 3-4 feet). Point your left foot to the left, and your right foot slightly to the left. Stretch your left arm out at shoulder level and bring the right arm straight up, against your right ear. Now inhale.*

2 *As you exhale, bend to the left and slightly forward to bypass your ribs. Slide your left hand down your left leg and hold on to the lowest part you can reach. Look out at your right hand. Take several full breaths in this position before releasing it. Repeat, bending to the right.*

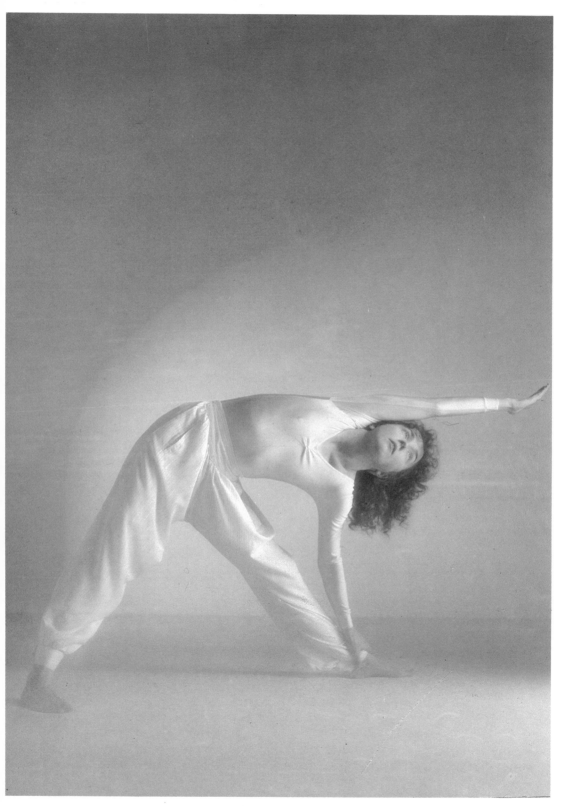

Basic Practice Charts

These charts are designed for easy reference, to help you to map your way through the Basic Session, whatever your level of experience. If you are a complete beginner, start by following the progressive 20-day course. This programme, divided into four 5-day periods, introduces you gently to the practice of yoga. For the first five days you concentrate solely on the exercises and asanas indicated in the first column, gradually building on this foundation during each of the following 5-day periods. We have not given any times for this "Basic Course", as students vary in their needs. Once you know the complete sequence, you can practise the "Typical

	Corpse Pose		Kapalabhati		Neck Rolls		Lion Pose		Leg Raises		Shoulderst	
	1	2	3	4	5	6	7	8	9	10	11	1
Phase 1	●	●	●*		●	●	●	●*	●			
Phase 2	●	●	●	●*	●	●	●	●*	●*		●*	
Phase 3	●	●	●	●*	●	●	●	●*	●*	●*	●*	
Phase 4	●	●	●	●*	●	●	●	●*	●*	●*	●*	
Half-Hour Class	1m		3m	4m*				5m*		3m*	1m*	½
Typical Class (1½ hours)	5m		4m	6m*	1m	2m	1m	10m*	5m	10m*	5m*	2
Pages	24	32	72	73	32	33	33	34	36	38	40	4

Basic Course: 4 phases, 5 days each

Key
m
minutes
*
corpse pose

Easy Pose   Anuloma Viloma   Eye Exercises   Sun Salutation   Headstand   Plough

Class", which takes about one and a half hours. Please note that the times given here indicate approximately how long you should spend working on a pose, not how long you should hold the final position. At every * in the sequence, relax in the Corpse Pose for at least six deep breaths. For those days when you are too short of time for a full session, we have included a "Half-Hour Class". This is a maintenance set of asanas which will keep your body tuned until you have time for a complete session. Whichever chart you are following, proceed systematically to make yoga a part of your daily routine. As Swami Sivananda says: "An ounce of practice is worth a ton of theory".

Bridge	Forward Bend		Locust		Half Spinal Twist		Crow		Triangle		
14	15	16	17	18	19	20	21	22	23	24	
									●		Phase 1
●*	●*	●*						●	●		Phase 2
●*	●*	●*		●*	●			●	●	●	Phase 3
●*	●*	●*	●*	●*	●	●	●	●	●	●	Phase 4
½m*	1m*	½m	½m*		1m			1m	1m	5m	Half-Hour Class
2½m*	5m*	2m*	2m*	2m*	2m	1m	1m*	2m	2m	10m	Typical Class (1½ hours)
46	48	50	52	54	56	58	60	62	64	24	

Basic Course: 4 phases, 5 days each

Fish   Cobra   Bow   Lotus   Hands to Feet   Corpse Pose

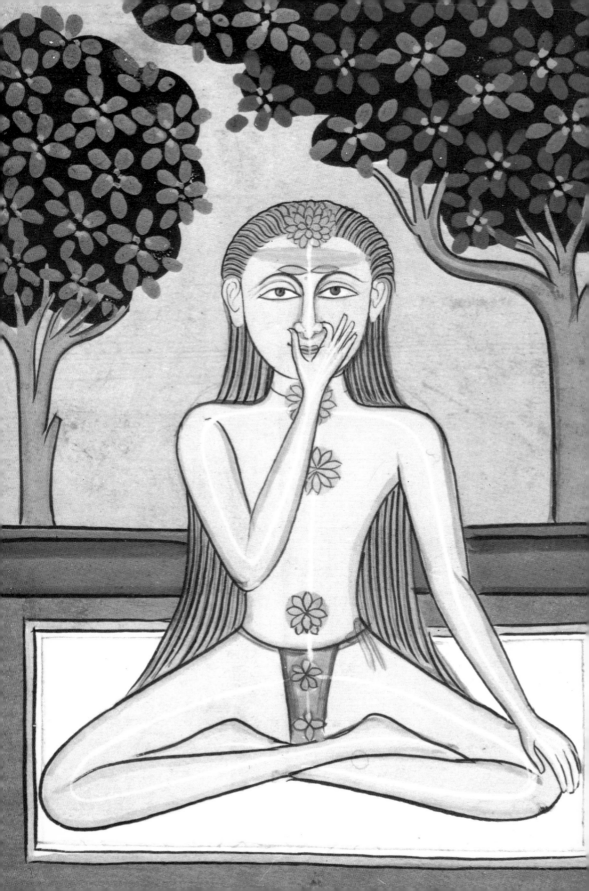

Breathing

"When the breath wanders, the mind is
unsteady, but when the breath is still, so is
the mind still."
Hatha Yoga Pradipika

Breath is life. We can live for days without food or water, but deprive us of breath and we die in minutes. In view of this, it is astonishing how little attention we pay in normal life to the importance of breathing correctly. To a yogi there are two main functions of proper breathing: to bring more oxygen to the blood and thus to the brain; and to control prana or vital energy (see p.70), leading to control of the mind. Pranayama – the science of breath control – consists of a series of exercises, especially intended to meet these needs and keep the body in vibrant health.

There are three basic types of breathing – clavicular (shallow), intercostal (middle) and abdominal breathing (deep). A full yogic breath combines all three, beginning with a deep breath and continuing the inhalation through the intercostal and clavicular areas.

Most people have forgotten how to breathe properly. They breathe shallowly, through the mouth, and make little or no use of the diaphragm – either lifting the shoulders or contracting the abdomen when they inhale. In this way, only a small amount of oxygen is taken in and only the top of the lungs used, resulting in lack of vitality and a low resistance to disease.

The practice of yoga demands that you reverse these habits. Breathing correctly means breathing through the nose, keeping the mouth closed, and involves a full inhalation and exhalation which bring the whole of your lungs into play. When you exhale, the abdomen contracts and the diaphragm moves up, massaging the heart; when you inhale, the abdomen expands and the diaphragm moves down, massaging the abdominal organs.

Just as there are three stages for an asana

(p.29), so in pranayama there are three parts to each breath – inhalation, retention, and exhalation. People often think of inhalation as the most essential stage of breathing but in fact it is exhalation that holds the key. For the more stale air you exhale, the more fresh air you can inhale (see p.182). The yogic breathing exercises lay special emphasis on a prolonged retention and exhalation – indeed in some exercises the outbreath is twice as long as the inbreath, and the retention four times as long.

When you inhale through your nose, the air is warmed and filtered. But from the yogic point of view the overriding reason for breathing nasally is prana. Just as you need to inhale through the nose to extract scents from the air, so you must also inhale nasally to maximize the amount of prana taken in – for at the back of the nose lie the olfactory organs through which prana passes to reach the central nervous system and brain.

The yoga breathing exercises teach you how to control prana and thus to control the mind, for the two are interdependent. When you are angry or scared, your breathing is shallow, rapid and irregular; conversely, when you are relaxed or deep in thought, your breathing becomes slow. You can easily test this yourself. Listen for a moment to the lowest sound in the room. You will find that, in concentrating, you unconsciously slowed down – or even suspended – your breathing.

Since your state of mind is reflected in the way you breathe, it follows that by controlling the breath you can learn to control your state of mind. By regulating your breathing you are thus not only increasing your intake of oxygen and prana, but preparing yourself for the practice of concentration and meditation.

Prana and the Subtle Body

Central to all the practices of yoga is the movement of prana, the life force or vital energy. Prana is in matter, but it is not matter. It is in air, but it is not oxygen. It is a subtle form of energy that is carried in air, food, water and sunlight, and animates all forms of matter. Through the practice of asanas and pranayama, more prana is taken in and stored in the body, bringing great vitality and strength. In addition to the physical body, yogis perceive man as possessing two other bodies that encircle it – the astral body and the causal body. Prana is the vital link between the astral and physical bodies, but it is mainly in the nadis of the astral body that it flows, as shown below. It exists both as a positive and a negative energy, when it is known as "apana". Prana itself is an afferent impulse, whose nature is to move upward; apana is efferent and moves downward. When the two are united at the Muladhara chakra, the Kundalini energy awakens.

Kundalini and the Nadis

The nadis are nerve channels or tubes in the astral body through which prana flows. Asanas and pranayama are designed to purify nadis, for when they are blocked prana cannot flow freely and poor health results. According to the ancient yogis, there are about seventy-two thousand nadis. Of all the nadis, the most important is the Sushumna, whose counterpart in the physical body is the spinal cord. On either side of the Sushumna, are two other nadis called Ida and Pingala, which correspond to the sympathetic ganglia of the spinal cord, as shown in the cross-section of a spinal vertebra, above right. Kundalini is a dormant or static cosmic energy, often depicted as a coiled snake. It is located at the base of the Sushumna in the Muladhara chakra and aroused or activated by pranayama and other yogic practices.

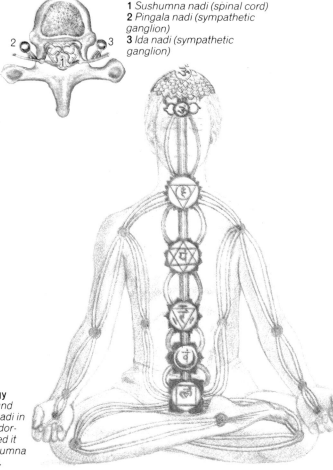

1 *Sushumna nadi (spinal cord)*
2 *Pingala nadi (sympathetic ganglion)*
3 *Ida nadi (sympathetic ganglion)*

The Path of Cosmic Energy
Ida and Pingala spiral around Sushumna, the principal nadi in the astral body. When the dormant Kundalini is awakened it starts to move up the Sushumna through the seven chakras.

The Seven Chakras

The chakras are centres of energy in the astral body. Six of them are located along the Sushumna; the seventh – the Sahasrara chakra – at the crown of the head. All are depicted with a certain number of petals, corresponding to the number of nadis emanating from them. Each petal represents a sound vibration produced when the Kundalini energy passes through the chakra. In addition, all the chakras except the Sahasrara have their own colour, element and bija mantra, as shown right, and all six correspond in the physical body to the nerve plexuses along the spine. At the base of the Sushumna is Muladhara, which corresponds to the sacral plexus. It is here that Kundalini lies dormant. Next is Swadhisthana, corresponding to the prostatic plexus. Manipura, the third chakra, corresponds to the solar plexus; it is the main storage centre for prana. Anahata – located in the region of the heart – corresponds to the cardiac plexus, Vishuddha – in the throat region – to the laryngeal plexus and Ajna chakra – located between the eyebrows – to the cavernous plexus.
Sahasrara, the seventh and highest chakra, corresponds in the physical body to the pineal gland. As Kundalini passes through each of the various chakras, different states of consciousness are experienced. When it reaches the Sahasrara, the yogi attains samadhi. Though still operating on the material plane, he has reached a level of existence beyond time, space and causation.

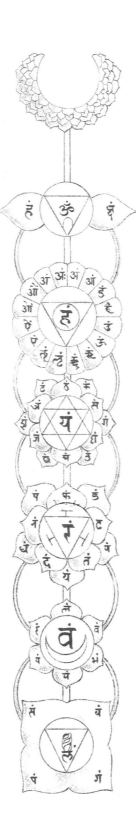

Sahasrara Chakra
The thousand-petalled crown chakra corresponds to the Absolute. When Kundalini reaches this point, the yogi attains samadhi or superconsciousness.

Ajna Chakra
This snow-white chakra has two petals. Seat of the mind, its mantra is OM.

Vishuddha Chakra
This sea-blue chakra has sixteen petals. Its element is ether and its mantra, Ham.

Anahata Chakra
This smoke-coloured chakra has twelve petals. Its element is air and its mantra, Yam.

Manipura Chakra
This red chakra has ten petals. Its element is fire and its mantra, Ram.

Swadhishthana Chakra
This white chakra has six petals. Its element is water and its mantra, Vam.

Muladhara Chakra
This yellow chakra has four petals. Its element is earth and its mantra, Lam.

Basic Breathing

Yogic breathing or pranayama revitalizes the body, steadies the emotions and creates great clarity of mind. Before practising the exercises, you should be sure that you understand how to breathe correctly, making full use of the diaphragm, as explained on page 69. In order to facilitate the flow of prana and ensure that there is space for expansion of the lungs, yoga breathing exercises are performed sitting down with the spine, neck and head in a straight line – either in the Easy Pose (p.32), the Lotus (p.58), or if neither of these is comfortable, sitting in a chair (p.172). Basic Breathing consists of five exercises. Kapalabhati and Anuloma Viloma are equivalent in importance to the Basic Session of asanas and should form the backbone of your pranayama. Practise them exclusively to begin with, before your daily set of asanas. Anuloma Viloma is the best exercise for purifying the nadis, and thus preparing the body for advanced pranayama. Brahmari, Sitkari, and Sithali are minor pranayamas which you can incorporate when you have time for a longer session.

"Pranayama is the link between the mental and physical disciplines. While the action is physical, the effect is to make the mind calm, lucid and steady."
Swami Vishnu Devananda

Kapalabhati

Kapalabhati is one of the six Kriyas or purification practices (p.154), besides being a pranayama. The forced exhalation rids the lower lungs of stale air, making way for a fresh intake of oxygen-rich air and cleansing the entire respiratory system. This is a wonderfully invigorating exercise to begin your pranayama. Translated literally its name means "skull shining" exercise and indeed, by increasing the amount of oxygen in the body, its effect is to clear the mind and improve the concentration. It consists of a series of exhalations and inhalations, followed by a retention of breath. To exhale you contract the abdominal muscles sharply, raising the diaphragm and forcing air out of the lungs; to inhale, you relax the muscles, allowing the lungs to fill with air. The exhalation should be brief, active and audible, the inhalation longer, passive and silent. The repeated up and down movement of the diaphragm tones the stomach, heart and liver. Begin by practising three rounds of twenty pumpings each and gradually work up to rounds of sixty.

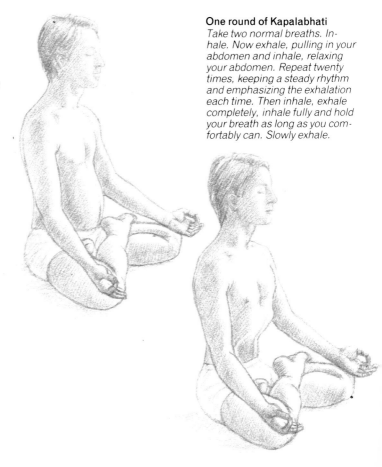

One round of Kapalabhati
Take two normal breaths. Inhale. Now exhale, pulling in your abdomen and inhale, relaxing your abdomen. Repeat twenty times, keeping a steady rhythm and emphasizing the exhalation each time. Then inhale, exhale completely, inhale fully and hold your breath as long as you comfortably can. Slowly exhale.

Anuloma Viloma

In this alternate nostril breathing exercise, you inhale through one nostril, retain the breath, then exhale through the other nostril in a ratio of 2:8:4. The left nostril is the path of the nadi called Ida, the right nostril that of Pingala. If you are really healthy, you will breathe predominantly through the Ida nostril for about one hour and fifty minutes, then through the Pingala nostril. But in many people this natural rhythm is disturbed. Anuloma Viloma restores an equal flow, balancing the flow of prana in the body. This is essential if you are to succeed in bringing prana up Sushumna, the central nadi (see p. 70). One round of Anuloma Viloma is made up of six steps, as shown below. Start by practising three rounds and build up slowly to twenty rounds, extending the count within the given ratio.

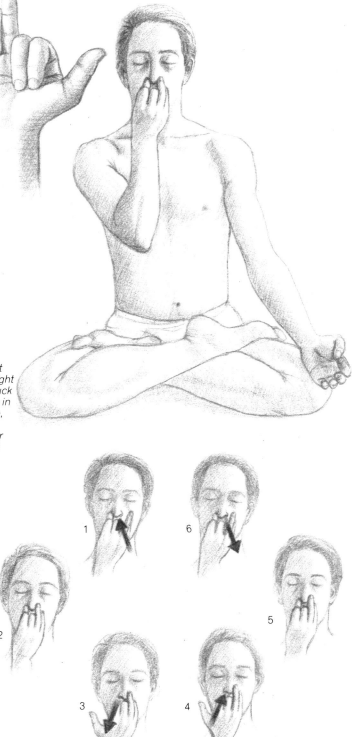

The Vishnu Mudra
In Anuloma Viloma, you adopt the Vishnu Mudra with your right hand to close your nostrils. Tuck your index and middle fingers in to your palm, as shown above, and raise your hand to your nose. Place the thumb by your right nostril and your ring and little fingers by your left. Now proceed as shown below.

One round of Anuloma Viloma
1 *Breathe in through the left nostril, closing the right with your thumb.*
2 *Hold the breath, closing both nostrils.*
3 *Breathe out through the right nostril, keeping the left nostril closed with your ring and little fingers.*
4 *Breathe in through the right nostril, keeping the left nostril closed.*
5 *Hold the breath, closing both nostrils.*
6 *Breathe out through the left nostril, keeping the right closed with your thumb.*

Brahmari

To practise Brahmari, you partially close the glottis as you inhale through both nostrils, making a snoring sound, then exhale slowly, humming like a bee. The inhalation clears and vibrates the throat area. Humming while you breathe out enables you to spin out the breath and make a longer exhalation. This extended exhalation makes it a very beneficial exercise for pregnant women, in preparation for labour. Sometimes known as the humming breath, Brahmari also gives a sweet clear voice and is highly recommended for singers. You should repeat Brahmari five to ten times.

Sitkari

Sitkari and Sithali (below) are unusual among yoga breathing exercises in that the inhalation is through the mouth rather than the nose. In Sitkari you press the tip of the tongue against the upper palate as you slowly inhale through the mouth, making a hissing sound. After retaining the breath as long as possible, you exhale slowly through the nose. Repeat five to ten times. Traditionally Sitkari is said to improve the countenance. The Hatha Yoga Pradipika prescribes: "By practising in this way, one becomes next to the God of Love in beauty." Both Sitkari and Sithali cool the body and relieve hunger and thirst. They are therefore particularly useful in hot weather or during a fast.

Sithali

Here you stick your tongue out a little way and curl the sides up, as shown right, making a "straw" to sip the air through as you inhale. Close the mouth while you hold the breath, then exhale slowly through the nose. If you are unable to curl your tongue round at first, just extend it slightly through your lips and sip in the air across its upper surface. Repeat five to ten times.

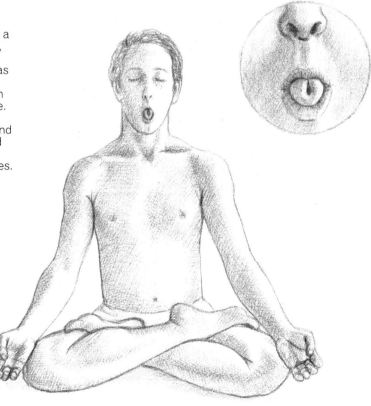

Advanced Breathing

Once you have been practising Kapalabhati and Anuloma Viloma for a few months and can perform them without effort or discomfort, you can start to think of expanding your pranayama session with these more advanced exercises. But first you should be sure that you are ready. The advanced pranayamas that follow are not to be taken lightly – they are powerful tools for controlling the flow of prana and raising the latent Kundalini energy. Before approaching them you should ideally have strengthened and purified yourself both physically and spiritually, by several months of daily asanas, pranayama and meditation and a wholesome vegetarian diet. Continue practising at least twenty rounds of Anuloma Viloma a day, in addition to these advanced exercises.

The Three Bandhas

Bandhas or "locks" are special postures that are adapted to conserve and make use of the vast reserves of prana generated by the Advanced Breathing exercises. They not only prevent the dissipation of prana, but also enable you to regulate its flow and convert it into spiritual energy. You should practise them separately for a few days before applying them in pranayama. Jalandhara and Moola Bandha are used simultaneously during retention to unite prana and apana (see p.70); Uddiyana Bandha is used after an exhalation to push the pranapana up into the Sushumna nadi, raising the Kundalini.

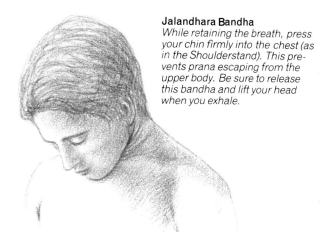

Jalandhara Bandha
While retaining the breath, press your chin firmly into the chest (as in the Shoulderstand). This prevents prana escaping from the upper body. Be sure to release this bandha and lift your head when you exhale.

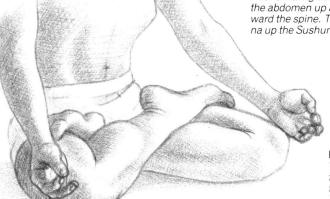

Uddiyana Bandha
After exhaling completely, pull the abdomen up and back toward the spine. This forces prana up the Sushumna nadi.

Moola Bandha
While retaining the breath, contract the anal sphincter muscle, then the abdominal muscles. This prevents apana escaping from the lower body and draws it up to unite with prana.

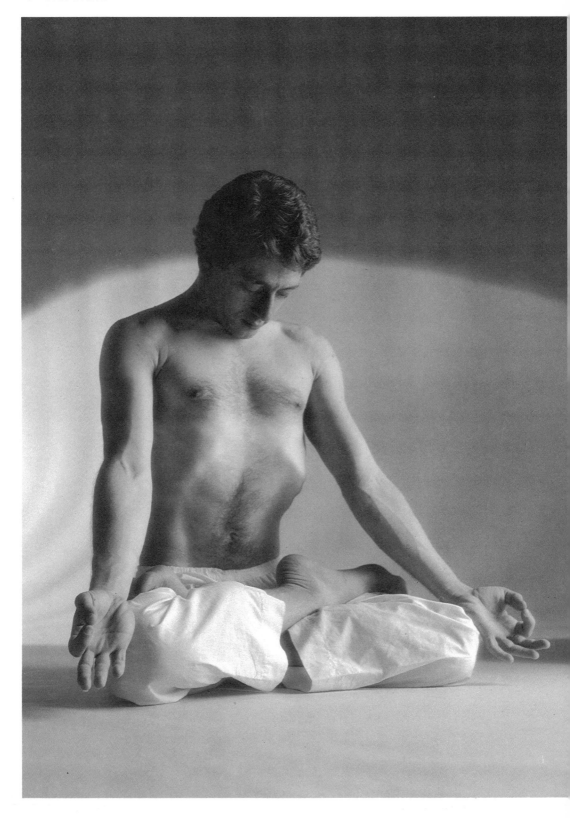

Ujjayi

Ujjayi strengthens the nervous and digestive systems and gets rid of phlegm. According to the ancient Yogic texts, disease is caused by an excess of either phlegm, wind or bile. Both Ujjayi and Surya Bheda are body-heating pranayamas and so exhalation is confined to the cooling left nostril, path of the nadi Ida. To practise Ujjayi, inhale fully through both nostrils while slightly closing the glottis (less than in Brahmari, page 74). This makes a faint sobbing sound, as the air is drawn past the back of your nose. Retain the breath, applying the Jalandhara and Moola Bandhas. Then release the two locks, close your right nostril with your right thumb and exhale through the left nostril. Start by practising five rounds at a sitting and increase gradually to twenty rounds.

Surya Bheda

In Surya Bheda, you inhale slowly through the right nostril, closing the left nostril with the ring and little fingers of your right hand; hold the breath, closing both nostrils and pressing your chin firmly against your chest in Jalandhara Bandha; then, keeping the right nostril closed with your thumb, exhale through the left nostril. You should gradually increase the period of retention. Surya means sun, referring to the right nostril, path of the Pingala nadi. When you inhale solely through this nostril, heat is created in the body and the impurities that impair the flow of prana are dispelled. Repeat Surya Bheda ten times at first and slowly build up to forty.

Bhastrika

This is the most powerful of all exercises for raising Kundalini. Bhastrika (which means "bellows") consists of a series of pumpings followed by a retention of breath like Kapalabhati. But there are important differences between the two: here you pump the lungs faster and more forcefully, using all the muscles of the respiratory system; you close both nostrils and apply Jalandhara and Moola Bandha while retaining the breath; and you exhale through the right nostril only, as during this exercise the body is heated, then cooled by perspiration. Then perform Uddiyana Bandha. Bhastrika is the best pranayama for the nervous and circulatory systems making the mind clear and focused. Start with three rounds of ten pumpings and work up slowly to a hundred pumpings and a maximum of eight rounds.

Samanu

Samanu is an advanced practice for purifying the nadis, that combines pranayama with chakra visualization and japa (p.98) on the bija mantras of air, fire, moon and earth.
1 Focusing on Anahata chakra, mentally repeat "yam" eight times while you inhale through the left nostril, 32 times while you retain, and sixteen times while you exhale through the right nostril.
2 Focusing on Manipura chakra, mentally repeat "ram", using the same ratio but inhaling through the right and exhaling through the left nostril.
3 Proceed as in 1, but focus on the moon centre at the tip of the nose and mentally repeat "tam" While you hold the breath, imagine the nectar of the moon suffusing the entire body. Exhale slowly, focusing on Muladhara chakra and repeating "lam".

Applying the Bandhas (left)
In Bhastrika, described above, you use all the bandhas to unite prana and apana and awaken the dormant Kundalini.

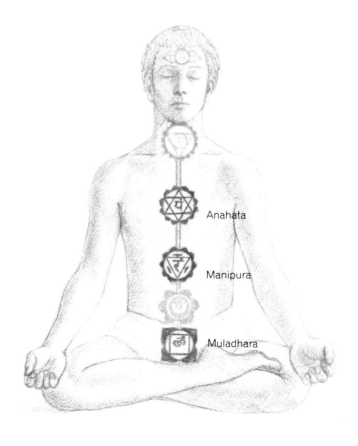

Anahata

Manipura

Muladhara

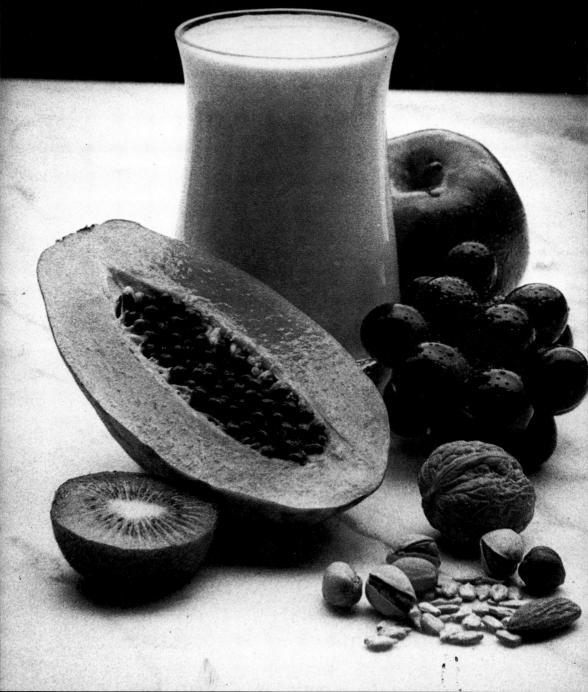

Diet

"Let the yogi eat moderately and abste-
miously; otherwise, however clever, he
cannot gain success."
Siva Samhita

We are what we eat. This statement is true in more senses than one. Food is of course necessary for our physical well-being. But as well as this it also has a subtle effect on our minds, since the essence of food forms the mind. A natural diet – a pure or "sattvic" one – is based on fresh, light, nutritional food such as fruit, grains and vegetables. It keeps the body lean and limber and the mind clear and sharp, making it most suitable for the practice of yoga. Full of prana, a pure and moderated diet is the best possible guarantee of physical and mental health, bringing harmony and vitality to both body and mind. In this section, we look at the reasons behind the yogic diet and give advice on how to change to a more balanced and wholesome eating pattern.

The yogic way of eating is quite simply the most natural. The sun, air, soil and water combine to produce the fruits of the earth – vegetables, fruit, legumes, nuts and seeds. The goodness we gain from these foods comes first hand. By contrast, the goodness obtained from eating meat, fish or poultry comes at second hand – we consume the flesh of creatures who have themselves pro-cessed the natural energy drawn from differ-ent plants. (It is interesting to note that we eat only herbivorous animals, such as cows, sheep and goats; only very exceptionally do we eat carnivorous creatures, such as dogs.) Animal flesh contains a high proportion of toxins (80 per cent of food poisoning cases are caused by meat or meat products) and tends to cause disease. It also lacks vital vitamins and minerals and contains more protein than we need. In eating meat, we are compelling our bodies to adapt to an unnatural diet, for which they are not designed. Our teeth and intestines are very different from those of carnivores – in fact, the anatomy and physiol-ogy of the fruit-eating primates is closest to our own.

But quite apart from the crucial considera-tions of health and natural goodness, meat-eating is both inefficient and wasteful. Many pounds of cereal must be fed to livestock to produce one pound of meat on the table; the "wasted" food is used to supply the animal with energy. As protein converters, livestock are inefficient. An acre of cereal will produce five times more protein than an acre devoted to raising animals for human consumption. The figures for legumes – ten times more – and leafy vegetables – fifteen times – are even more startling. Some individual vegetables are yet more efficient.

In establishing a natural diet, we must also ask ourselves whether we can consume with a clear conscience the flesh of a living creature, of another being slaughtered often under the most barbaric conditions. In the so-called civilized world we are distanced and anaesthetized from the horrors of the meat industry. Faced with neatly packaged portions of meat or fish we no longer make the connection between the product and the animal that has been killed – unnecessarily for our sakes. Ahimsa – the sanctity of all living creatures – is among the highest laws in yogic philosophy and cannot be disregarded if we are to grow spiritually. For the yogi, all life is sacred: every creature is a living entity, with a heart and emotions, breathing and feeling, so even to contemplate eating meat or fish is quite impossible. Once you become con-scious of where your food comes from and how it affects you, your mind will gradually open, and you will come to realise that all creatures are as divine as you yourself are.

The Three Gunas

In the unmanifested Universe, energy has three qualities, known as Gunas, that exist together in equilibrium: Sattva (purity); Rajas (activity, passion, the process of change); and Tamas (darkness, inertia). Once energy takes form, one quality of the three predominates (see p.18). Thus on an apple tree, some of the fruit is ripe (sattvic), some ripening (rajasic) and some overripe (tamasic). But no matter which quality prevails, an element of each of the other two will always be present as well. Most of an individual apple will be ripe, but part will be rotten, even if the naked eye cannot see it, and part will be in the process of changing from one state to the other. The three Gunas encompass all existence, all actions. If a man commits a robbery, the action is basically rajasic but the decision to rob and the motive may be predominantly tamasic, rajasic or sattvic, according to the situation. In all men one of the three Gunas has superior strength and is reflected in all they do and think. Only in enlightenment are the Gunas completely transcended.

Beyond the Three Gunas (right)
Only the enlightened Self, the state of consciousness known as samadhi, transcends the three Gunas. In this picture, all the other elements – the man's body and mind, the tree and the steps – are subject to the Gunas.

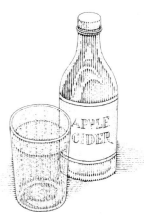

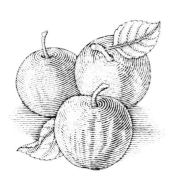

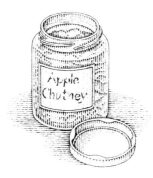

Sattvic Food

This is the purest diet, the most suitable one for any serious student of yoga. It nourishes the body and maintains it in a peaceful state. And it calms and purifies the mind, enabling it to function at its maximum potential. A sattvic diet thus leads to true health: a peaceful mind in control of a fit body, with a balanced flow of energy between them. Sattvic foods include cereals, wholemeal bread, fresh fruit and vegetables, pure fruit juices, milk, butter and cheese, legumes, nuts, seeds, sprouted seeds, honey, and herb teas.

Rajasic Food

Foods that are very hot, bitter, sour, dry or salty are rajasic. They destroy the mind–body equilibrium, feeding the body at the expense of the mind. Too much rajasic food will over-stimulate the body and excite the passions, making the mind restless and uncontrollable. Rajasic foods include hot substances, such as sharp spices or strong herbs, stimulants, like coffee and tea, fish, eggs, salt, and chocolate. Eating in a hurry is also considered rajasic.

Tamasic Food

A tamasic diet benefits neither the mind nor the body. Prana, or energy, is withdrawn, powers of reasoning become clouded and a sense of inertia sets in. The body's resistance to disease is destroyed and the mind filled with dark emotions, such as anger and greed. Tamasic items include meat, alcohol, tobacco, onions, garlic, fermented foods, such as vinegar, and stale or overripe substances. Overeating is also regarded as tamasic.

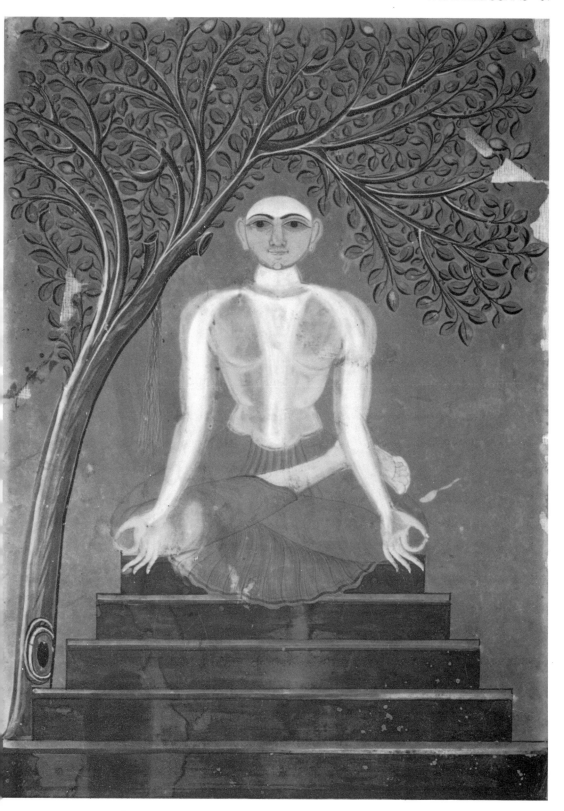

Natural Foods

Until quite recently most meat-eaters viewed vegetarians with a certain suspicion, dismissing them as cranks or food faddists who lived on an unappetizing diet of brown rice and nut cutlets. Nowadays, people are better informed, but the vegetarian diet is still sometimes dismissed as dull and uninteresting, and lacking in vital nutrients. The facts show quite the reverse – indeed, if anyone needs to defend that accusation it is meat-eaters. There is ample medical evidence that a balanced vegetarian diet is extremely healthy, and provides all the protein, minerals and so on that the body requires. Statistically, vegetarians have a lower incidence of heart attacks, strokes, kidney disease, and cancer; their

The Protein Question

Fear of protein deficiency is the meat-eater's main objection to a vegetarian diet. Yet, ironically, meat-eaters themselves obtain the worst quality protein from their food – protein that is dead or dying. We ourselves are animals, and can take our protein from the plant world, just as well as other herbivorous animals. Animal protein contains too much uric acid to be broken down by the liver; some is eliminated, but the rest is deposited in the joints, causing stiffness and eventually leading to problems like arthritis. Nuts, dairy produce, spirulina, and legumes – especially the soya bean and its products, such as tofu and soya milk – all supply high-class protein. Westerners are obsessed with protein, believing that they need far more than they actually do. In fact there is considerable disagreement between the various scientific bodies as to the exact daily protein requirements. The World Health Organization presently recommends a daily intake of 25 to 50 grams as sufficient to maintain and replace body tissue.

Complementary Foods

More important than the quantity of protein we consume is its quality. Proteins are made up of amino acids, some of which can by synthesized by the body. But others must be included in the diet. The key to a well-balanced amino-acid content in the diet is the combination of complementary foods. To get the maximum value from your food as a vegetarian you should set out to build complete protein meals. Some basic combinations are: cereals (wholemeal bread, rice, etc.) with legumes (beans, peas and lentils); cereals with dairy products; and seeds (sesame or sunflower) with legumes. Three classically simple meals can serve as examples of this principle – cereals and milk, bread and cheese, and rice with beans. Meals constructed on these lines will give the body all the protein it requires. They are also appetizing, require very little preparation, and offer the inventive cook an endless variety of menus. This is fresh, natural food at its best.

Fat and Fibre

A vegetarian diet is also full of fibre and rich in polyunsaturated fats. Lack of dietary fibre, which is contained in unrefined plant food, leads to a number of disorders of the intestine. Research in southern England has shown that vegetarians consume almost twice as much fibre as meat-eaters. They also consume less fat; and the fats they do eat tend to be polyunsaturated and not the saturated animal fats that raise blood cholesterol.

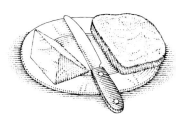

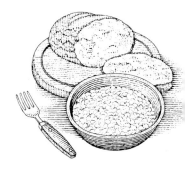

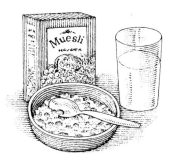

Complete Protein Meals
Simple vegetarian meals, well-balanced in protein, include wholemeal bread and cheese or beans – as stew or salad – and cereals with milk.

resistance to disease is higher; and they are less likely to suffer from obesity than meat-eaters. The choice of fruits, vegetables, legumes, nuts, seeds and cereals is abundant. And these foods can be prepared in a multitude of different ways, offering an enormous range of tastes and textures. To keep the body healthy, your diet should include each of the elements shown in the chart below, as well as water. Carbohydrates and fats are the energy-giving foods, proteins, vitamins and minerals the essential body-building materials. The exact requirements vary from person to person. Active people, for example, need more carbohydrates and fats, children and pregnant women more protein and calcium.

Chart of Food Values
The analysis of a few common foods reveals surprisingly different values. For example, nuts and cheese are very high in protein, bread high in minerals.

Key

Na	Sodium
K	Potassium
Ca	Calcium
Mg	Magnesium
P	Phosphorus
S	Sulphur
Cl	Chloride

Foods (100g)	Proteins (g)	Carbo hydrates(g)	Fats (g)	Minerals (over 10mg)	Vitamins (over 10mg)
Apples	0.3	11.9	—	K	A
Bananas	0.7	11.4	0.2	K Mg P Cl	B
Oranges	0.6	6.2	–	K Ca Mg P	A, C
Cabbage, raw	1.9	3.8	–	K Ca Mg P	B, C
Potatoes, baked	2.6	25.0	0.1	K Mg P S Cl	B, C
Tomatoes	0.9	2.8	–	K Mg P S Cl	A, B, C
Lentils	7.6	17.0	0.5	Na K Ca Mg P S	B
Peas	5.8	10.6	0.4	K Ca Mg P S Cl	A, B, C
Bread, wholemeal	0.7	41.8	2.7	Na K Ca Mg P S Cl	B
Pasta	4.2	26.0	0.3	K Mg P S Cl	–
Rice	2.2	29.6	0.3	K P S	B
Butter	0.4	–	82.0	Na K Ca P Cl	A
Cheese, cheddar	26.0	–	33.5	Na K Ca Mg P S Cl	A
Milk, whole	3.3	4.7	3.8	Na K Ca Mg P S Cl	A
Yoghurt, plain	5.0	6.2	1.0	Na K Ca Mg P Cl	–
Nuts (almonds)	16.9	4.3	53.5	K Ca Mg P S	A, B
Margarine, vegetable	0.1	0.1	81.0	Na P S Cl	–
Honey	0.4	76.4	–	Na K P Cl	–

Changing your Diet

Becoming a vegetarian is a positive step. You are not just deciding to stop eating meat, you are opening the door to a new way of life. For some the changeover is easy; for others it may take a little longer. It is best to change your diet gradually rather than dramatically, slowly phasing out meat and fish and substituting well-balanced vegetarian foods. You will soon find that your desire to eat meat grows weaker. It will help if you spend some time researching the whole subject. Read up on how to balance your diet and on the drawbacks and hazards of meat-eating. If you are mentally committed to the concept of vegetarianism, it will be far easier to make the switch. In addition to giving up meat and fish, anyone seriously interested in yoga should phase out eggs, alcohol, cigarettes, coffee, tea and other drugs. People sometimes worry that eating out will be a problem if they become vegetarians. But over the last ten years, more and more vegetarian restaurants have sprung up – and even in those that do not cater specifically for you, there is nearly always something that you can happily eat. A purer diet will make it easier for you to do asanas – for the less meat you eat, the less stiff your body will be. And just as a more sattvic diet will help in your practice of yoga, so by the regular practice of asanas, pranayama and meditation, your consciousness will change and rajasic or tamasic foods will start to lose their appeal.

"Every herb bearing seed . . . and every tree in which is the fruit of a tree yielding seed; to you they shall be for meat."
Genesis 1:29

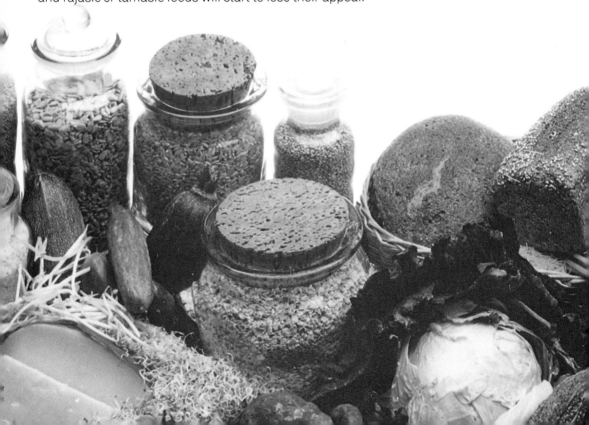

Here are a few hints to ease the changeover.
1 Ensure that you have a regular intake of good protein foods, such as nuts, pulses, whole grains, and cheese.
2 Eat a salad of raw vegetables each day – cut or grate some and leave others whole, to give you a variety of textures.
3 Include plenty of green, leafy vegetables in your diet.
4 If you are cooking vegetables, do so as quickly as possible, in order to preserve their goodness. Steaming or stir-frying are the best methods.
5 Eat some fresh fruit every day. If you cook fruit, do so rapidly – long, slow cooking destroys a lot of the vitamins.
6 Take care that the food you eat is fresh and wholesome: stale nuts, wrinkled, rotten fruit and limp greens become tamasic and lose much of their original food value.
7 Avoid "denatured" foods, such as white flour, white bread, cakes, refined cereals, canned fruit, vegetables and drinks, and saturated fats, such as hydrogenized oils.
8 Cook only as much as you are going to eat and no more. Reheating food kills much of its nutritional value.
9 Be inventive and adventurous – introduce variety into your diet by experimenting with new ingredients.
10 Learn to substitute more sattvic foods for rajasic or tamasic ones – use tofu instead of eggs, for instance, honey for sugar, herb teas for black tea.

"By the purity of food, follows the purification of the inner nature."
Swami Sivananda

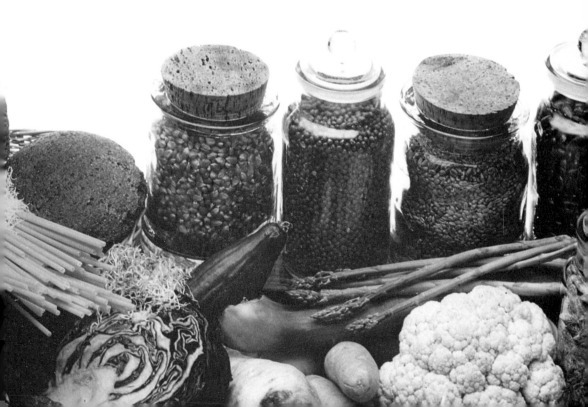

Fasting

As a means of purification and self-disclipine, fasting stretches way back in time. The early American Indians fasted to see the Great Spirit, Christ spent forty days and forty nights in the wilderness, and Moses fasted on Mount Sinai. Yogis fast mainly to bring the mind and senses under control, but also to cleanse and thus rejuvenate the body. In fact, fasting is the body's natural way of dealing with illness or pain – animals in the wild will stop eating when hurt or unwell and we ourselves lose our appetites if we are feverish. In normal life, much of our energy is devoted to the process of digestion. Resting the digestive system releases this energy for spiritual development and for self-healing, allowing the body to rid itself of toxins. On no account should fasting be confused with dieting. Its purpose is to purify the body and mind, not to lose weight – indeed, some people actually gain weight after a fast.

How to Fast

First you must resolve when and for how long you want to fast. Choose a time when you are not too busy and are not taking any kind of medication – a fast is a form of medicine in its own right. Fasting one day a week is a good discipline to strengthen your will power, but you will need more time if you want to detoxify the system. Fasts of four days can be safely undertaken without supervision, but not longer. Decide what kind of fast you are going to follow – water, fruit juice or vegetable juice – and stick to it exclusively. On a water fast, drink five to seven glasses of pure bottled or spring water a day – drink them slowly so as to absorb the prana. On a juice fast, drink the same amount, but "chew" the juice rather than simply swallowing it. Enemas and kriyas will speed up the cleansing process, especially at the beginning of a fast. Enemas or Basti (p. 153) remove waste from the intestines, while Kunjar Kriya is useful on the first day of fasting to get rid of toxins from the base of the stomach. Drink four glasses of lukewarm water, each with a teaspoon of salt. Then contract your stomach and put two fingers down your throat until you bring all the water up.

The first three days of fasting are the hardest. As the body strives to rid itself of impurities, you may experience any of the following effects: headaches; a coated tongue; bad breath; and vomiting. If you have palpitations, take fruit juice if you are on a water fast, fruit in on a juice fast. Breathing difficulties also sometimes occur, but can usually be overcome by pranayama. If either the palpitations or the breathing problems persist, break the fast slowly. Fasting slows down the circulation, so you need to wear more clothes than usual to keep warm and may experience a little dizziness if you move too quickly or suddenly. During a fast, many impurities are dispersed through the skin, so don't use make-up or anti-perspirants which block the pores. You should learn to

Breaking the Fast

Perhaps the most difficult part of a fast is breaking it sensibly, for as soon as you taste food your mind will demand that you eat and eat. But just as, having slept, you don't want to wake up to a barrage of questions, so after fasting, you must re-accustom your body gradually to eating, choosing your first food with care. To make sure that you don't overindulge to begin with, break your fast in the evening and do not eat again until this food has gone through the system. Vegetarians should take about a pound of fresh fruit – grapes (without seeds), cherries, or other juicy fruits, but not bananas, apples or citrus fruits. People whose diet has been heavier, such as meat-eaters, should have the same amount of steamed spinach or stewed tomatoes. Then, for a two-day fast, proceed as follows:

On Day 1 – fresh fruit only as above, plus a teaspoon of natural yoghurt to aid digestion.
On Day 2 – take only salads.
On Day 3 – steamed vegetables with light grain, such as buckwheat or millet.
On Day 4 – return gradually to your normal diet.

If you fasted for four days, simply double the above timetable, allowing yourself two days on fresh fruit alone and so on. Tea, coffee, alcohol and seasonings should be avoided while breaking a fast, and an enema taken on days 1 and 3.
Try to stick closely to this regime, so as not to over-burden the system. As George Bernard Shaw said: "Any fool can go on a fast, but it takes a wise man to break it properly."

conserve your energy while fasting – go for a quiet walk every day but avoid strenuous exercise, such as jogging. Practise at least one set of asanas and breathing exercises each day, to break up the accumulated toxins and hasten their removal from the body. And allow some time for meditation – your mind will be far steadier during a fast. After a few days your stomach will no longer crave food and you will begin to notice some of the benefits – an enhanced sense of smell, for example, and increased mental energy and concentration. Abstaining from eating gives you a chance to devote more time to your spiritual development and to realise the extent to which you can control your own patterns of thinking, behaving, eating and so on. In order not to waste what you have learnt, it is important that you break the fast wisely and systematically, as described opposite.

The Middle Way

Shakyamuni lived many years as a wandering ascetic, going without food or water until he was reduced to skin and bone. At last, weary of these exertions, he took food and sat under a pipal tree, vowing not to move until he had found Enlightenment. All night long he was plagued with demons, but as day broke he achieved his goal and attained Nirvana. As Buddha, he went on to preach the wisdom of the middle path, between the extremes of indulgence and self-mortification.

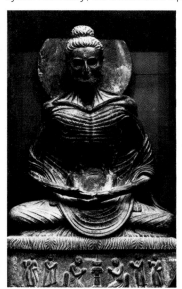

Fasting Buddha in Meditation *(above), a 19th-century sculpture from North India.*

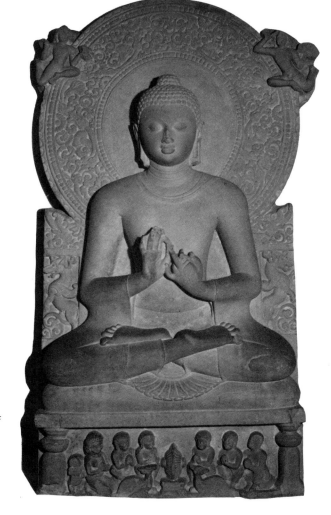

The Enlightened One *(right) a renowned 5th-century image of Buddha from Sarnath, India.*

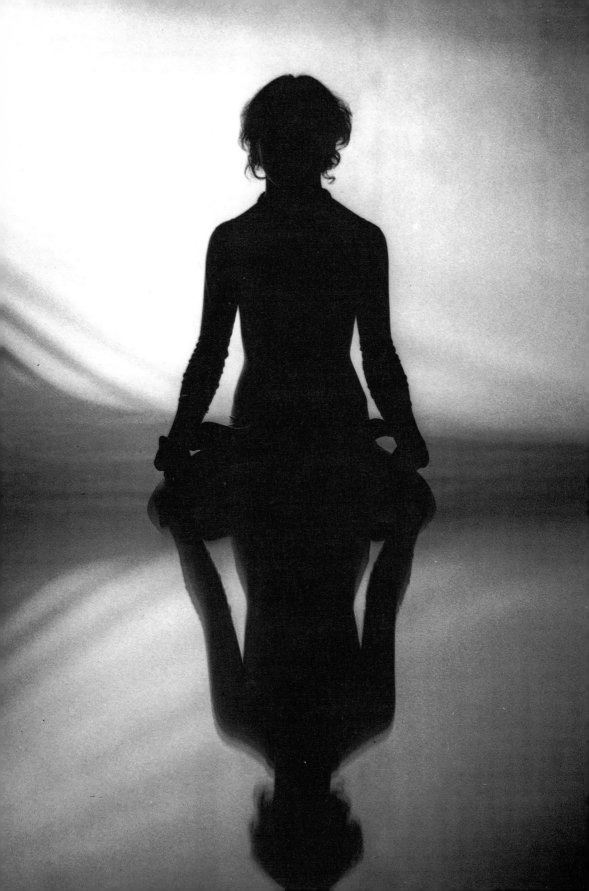

Meditation

"Meditation is a continuous flow of
perception or thought, like the
flow of water in a river."
Swami Vishnu Devananda

Consciously or unconsciously we are all
seeking the peace of mind that meditation
brings. All of us have our own ways of finding
this peace, our own meditative habits – from
the old lady who sits knitting by the fire to the
boatman whiling away a summer's afternoon
by the river, oblivious to the passing of time.
For when our attention is fully engaged, the
mind becomes silent; when we succeed in
restricting our thoughts to one object, the
incessant internal chattering stops. Indeed
the contentment we feel when our minds are
absorbed often comes less from the activity
itself than from the fact that in concentrating,
our worries or problems are forgotten.

But these activities can only bring us a
short interlude of peace for as long as they
absorb our interest. Once the mind is again
distracted, it returns to its normal routine of
aimless wandering – wasting its energy on
thoughts of the past or dreams of the future,
continually sidestepping the matter at hand.
To find a more lasting contentment, you need
to train the mind in meditation.

Meditation is the practice by which there is
constant observation of the mind. It means
focusing the mind on one point, stilling the
mind in order to perceive the Self. By stopping the waves of thoughts you come to
understand your true nature and discover the
wisdom and tranquillity that lie within.

Focusing on the flame of a candle, say, or
on a mantra (p.98), you repeatedly bring your
attention back to the object of concentration,
reducing the movement of the mind to a small
circle. At first your thoughts will insist on
wandering; but with steady practice you will
succeed in extending the time the mind is
focused. In the beginning, while your attention still wavers, meditation is more properly

called concentration; in meditation, you
achieve an unbroken flow of thoughts. The
difference between the two is one of degree,
not of technique. Swami Vishnu explains it
this way: "During concentration, one keeps a
tight rein on the mind; during meditation, the
rein is no longer necessary, for the mind stays
of its own accord on one single thought
wave."

In Patanjali's Eight Limbs, concentration
and meditation are the sixth and seventh
steps of Raja Yoga (see p.16). The eighth is
samadhi or superconsciousness, a state
beyond time, space and causation where
body and mind are transcended and total
unity exists. In samadhi, the meditator and
the object of concentration become one – for
it is the ego that creates a sense of separation
or duality. According to the ancient Vedas,
concentration or dharana is fixing the mind
on one thought for twelve seconds; meditation or dhyana is equal to twelve dharanas –
about two and a half minutes – and samadhi
to twelve dhyanas – just under half an hour.

In the same way that focusing the rays of
the sun with a magnifying glass makes them
hot enough to burn, just so focusing the
scattered rays of thought makes the mind
penetrating and powerful. With the continued
practice of meditation, you discover a greater
sense of purpose and strength of will and
your thinking becomes clearer and more
concentrated, affecting all you do.

As Swami Vishnu has written: "Meditation
does not come easily. A beautiful tree grows
slowly. One must wait for the blossom, the
ripening of the fruit and the ultimate taste.
The blossom of meditation is an expressible
peace that permeates the entire being. Its
fruit . . . is undescribable."

Mastery of the Mind

The mind is like a lake, its surface broken by ripples of thought. In order to see the Self which lies beneath, first you must learn to still these ripples, to become the master of your mind rather than its servant. For most of your waking hours the mind is tossed from one thought to another, pulled by desires and aversions, by emotions and memories, both pleasant and unpleasant. Of all the forces that agitate the mind it is the senses that most often disturb the concentration, giving rise to fantasies and desires. A well-loved tune on the radio sends the mind racing to the time you heard it first, while a tempting smell or a sudden cold draught can shatter your train of thought. Of all the senses, sight and hearing are the most powerful, endlessly drawing the mind outward and wasting valuable mental energy. For this reason meditation uses either sounds (mantras) or images (in Tratak).

The mind is by by nature constantly searching for happiness, vainly hoping to find satisfaction once it attains what it desires. On acquiring the desired object, the mind is temporarily silenced, but after a short while the whole pattern starts again, because the mind itself remains unchanged and the true desire unfulfilled. Imagine, for example, that you go out and buy a new car. For some time you feel proud and satisfied – the mind is at rest. But soon you start hankering after a newer model or a different colour, or worrying about it getting stolen or hit. What began as a pleasure has become yet another source of discontent, for in stilling one desire, many others are created.

Yoga teaches us that we possess a source of joy and wisdom already inside us, a fund of tranquillity that we can perceive and draw nourishment from when the movement of the mind is still. If we can channel this desire for contentment inward instead of attaching it to external objects that are by nature ephemeral, we can discover how to live in peace.

Witnessing the Play of Thoughts

During meditation you experience the mind as an instrument. Just by concentrating for a short period each day, you start to see how much movement exists in the mind, and how little you live in the present. From this brief encounter with a different mode of perception, you can learn to observe and thus change your way of thinking. One of the most useful tools for controlling the mind is to stop associating with your emotions, thoughts and actions. Instead of identifying with them, you simply step back and assume the role of witness, as if you were watching someone else. By observing yourself dispassionately in this way, without judgment or praise, your thoughts and emotions lose their power over you – you start to see both mind and body as instruments that you can control. In detaching from the games of the ego, you learn to take responsibility for yourself.

"Just as the beauty and sweet fragrance of the Lotus flower are only revealed when it rises up from the muddy water and turns toward the sun, so our lives will only grow in beauty when we leave behind the world of Maya or illusion and look toward God, through meditation".
Swami Vishnu Devananda

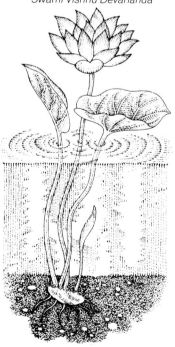

Meditation in Daily Life

You are unlikely to succeed in taming the mind in your brief session of meditation if you allow it free rein the rest of the time. The longer you spend with the mind concentrated, the sooner you will be able to focus when you sit down to meditate. Apart from the meditation techniques given on the following pages, there is much that you can do to keep your mind centered. While walking, for example, try to synchronize your breathing with your footsteps – inhale for three steps, exhale for three. Breathing slowly and with control quietens the mind down too (see p.69). When reading a book, test your concentration by stopping at the end of a page to see how much you can remember. And don't restrict japa to your session of meditation – repeat your mantra on the way to work, for example, while doing your asanas or preparing a meal. Most important of all, keep your thinking as positive as possible. On days where your peace of mind is shattered by anger or unhappiness, you can often calm yourself by focusing on the opposite emotion – countering feelings of hatred with love, for example, doubt with faith or hope. By using these simple techniques you will slowly accustom your mind to a state of concentration. You will begin to notice that external influences are having less effect on you. Whether you have a difficult week at the office or an enjoyable day out in the country, your mood remains the same, for your inner core is growing stronger. You gain the security of knowing that in the midst of the changes that are life's essence, you can remain constant and assured.

The Types of Meditation

In yoga there are two main types of meditation – concrete or Saguna (literally "with qualities") and abstract or Nirguna (without qualities). In Saguna meditation you focus on a concrete object on which the mind can easily dwell – on an image or visual symbol, perhaps, or a mantra which brings you to unity. In Nirguna meditation, the point of focus is an abstract idea, such as the Absolute, a concept that is indescribable in words. Saguna meditation is dualistic – the meditator considers himself separate from the object of meditation, whereas in Nirguna meditation the meditator perceives himself as one with the object. The techniques of meditation given in this section are predominantly Saguna, since even though your concept of the Absolute may be abstract, it is harder to hold the mind to an abstract concept. But for those of you who can, we have included two Nirguna mantras (p.99) – Om and Soham. Regardless of whether you practise Saguna or Nirguna meditation, the end is ultimately the same – transcendence of the Gunas. As Swami Vishnu says in his teachings: "The purpose of life is to fix the mind on the Absolute".

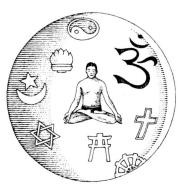

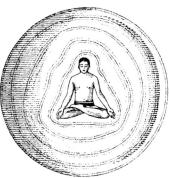

Saguna and Nirguna Meditation
Imagine yourself sitting in the centre of a sphere which repre-sents the Absolute. In Saguna meditation (top) you focus on and become one with a symbol on the sphere's surface, such as OM (p.96) or the Cross. In Nirgu-na meditation (above) you don't identify with any of the symbols or aspects of the Absolute. Your awareness expands to encom-pass and merge with the sphere itself.

The Principles of Meditation

Meditation, like sleep, cannot be taught – it comes by itself, in its own time. But if you follow the right steps to begin with, you can speed up your progress considerably. To help people to understand the basic steps and stages of meditation, Swami Vishnu formulated the Twelve Principles, summarized right. The most essential thing is to establish meditation as a regular habit in your life, using the same place and time each day. This will train your mind to respond without delay once you sit down to meditate – much as your stomach is conditioned to expect food at mealtimes. After a few months of regular practice, your mind will begin to demand this quiet time of its own accord. The most auspicious times of day for meditation are at dawn and at dusk, when the atmosphere is charged with spiritual energy. But if neither of these times is possible, simply choose a time when you can be alone and undisturbed. Start by practising for twenty minutes, and gradually increase the time to an hour. Sit facing the East or North to benefit from the subtle effects of the earth's magnetic field. You may want to wrap a blanket around yourself before you start so as to keep warm. It is most important that your sitting position is steady and relaxed, as your concentration will be disturbed if you are uncomfortable. Before beginning, instruct your mind to be silent and to forget all thoughts of the past, present or future. Now regulate your breathing – this will control the flow of prana which in turn will help to still the mind. You should not attempt to combat the restlessness of your mind, as this will only generate more thought waves. Simply detach yourself from your thoughts and watch your mind .

"The Self is not the individual body or mind, but rather that aspect deep inside each person that knows the Truth."
Swami Vishnu Devananda

The Twelve Principles
1 *Set aside a special place for meditation – the atmosphere you build up will help still the mind.*
2 *Choose a time when your mind is free of everyday concerns – dawn and dusk are ideal.*
3 *Using the same time and place each day conditions the mind to slow down more quickly.*
4 *Sit with your back, neck and head in a straight line, facing North or East.*
5 *Instruct your mind to remain quiet for the duration of your meditation session.*
6 *Regulate your breathing – start with five minutes' deep breathing, then slow it down.*
7 *Establish a rhythmic breathing pattern – inhaling then exhaling for about three seconds.*
8 *At first, let your mind wander – it will only grow more restless if you force it to concentrate.*
9 *Now bring the mind to rest on the focal point of your choice – either the Ajna or the Anahata chakra (p. 71).*
10 *Applying your chosen technique, hold your object of concentration at this focal point throughout your session.*
11 *Meditation comes when you reach a state of pure thought, but still retain your awareness of duality.*
12 *After long practice, duality disappears and samadhi, the superconscious state, is attained.*

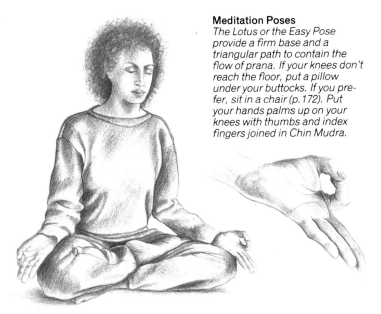

Meditation Poses
The Lotus or the Easy Pose provide a firm base and a triangular path to contain the flow of prana. If your knees don't reach the floor, put a pillow under your buttocks. If you prefer, sit in a chair (p. 172). Put your hands palms up on your knees with thumbs and index fingers joined in Chin Mudra.

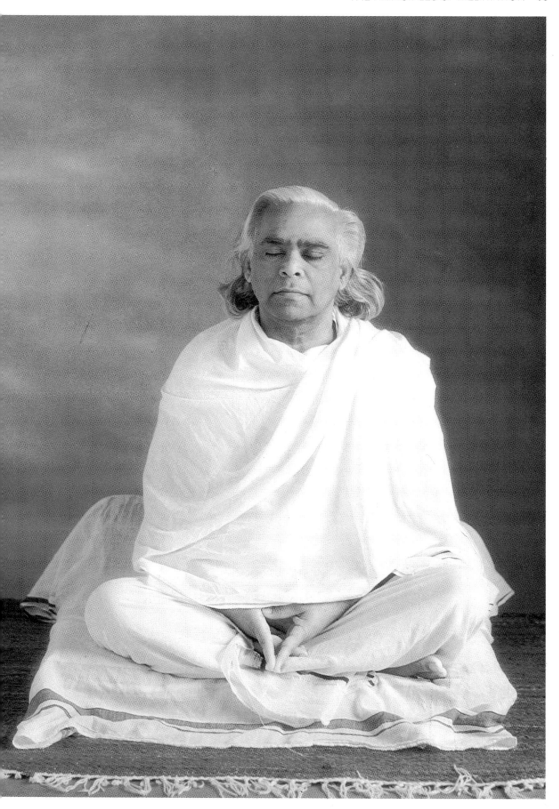

Starting to Meditate

In the long tradition of meditation, there is a great variety of different techniques – some using the power of sound, others using visual symbols or breathing. But all have a common aim: to focus the scattered rays of the mind on a single point, so as to lead the meditator to a state of self-realization. The technique that we recommend most highly for long-term practice is japa – repeating a mantra, as described on page 98. But if you are a newcomer to meditation, you may wish to make use of another technique in addition to using a mantra, to help to discipline your mind at first.

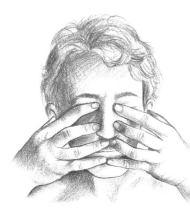

Yoni Mudra

Yoni Mudra is an exercise in pratyahara or withdrawal of the senses. Blocking off your ears, eyes, nose and mouth you retreat inside yourself, like a tortoise drawing its legs in under its shell. During the day the mind is constantly bombarded with information and stimuli from the five senses. Only when the senses are brought under control and the mind is no longer pulled constantly outward, can you hope to be able to concentrate. You will already have had a foretaste of how it feels to shut off one of the senses by practising asanas on an empty stomach – and perhaps, also, with eyes closed. By allowing you to rest undisturbed inside your mind, Yoni Mudra makes you more fully aware of the tyranny of the senses. It is a technique that you can return to whenever you feel particularly restless or agitated. As your concentration deepens, you will begin to hear the anahata or mystic inner sounds while practising it – sounds like flutes, drums, or bells for example, signals of a heightened awareness. The Siva Samhita, one of the yogic texts, says of Yoni Mudra: "The Yogi, by having thus firmly confined the air, sees his soul in the shape of light."

Yoni Mudra
Close your ears with your thumbs. Cover your eyes with your index fingers, then close your nostrils with your middle fingers and press your lips together with your remaining fingers. Release the middle fingers gently to inhale and exhale while you meditate.

Category Concentration

When learning to meditate it is hard to keep your attention focused on one object to start with. To train yourself to pay attention you can try narrowing your field of concentration to a category of objects first, where your mind still has a little freedom of movement. In the category concentration exercise, shown below right, you choose four flowers as objects of concentration. After concentrating on one, you can move on to the next when your mind starts to wander. If you don't feel at ease concentrating on flowers, choose a different category of objects, such as fruit or trees. It is only important that you restrict your mind to a group of objects and that the objects you choose are ones you can regard with detachment. Practising this exercise will hone your mind down to a finer focus and teach you the principle of one-pointed concentration. Once you find no difficulty in visualizing and remaining focused on a category of objects you are ready to move on to concentrate on one single object.

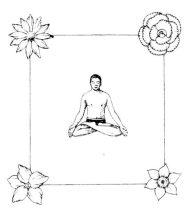

Category Concentration
With eyes closed, imagine a garden with a different flower in each corner. Start by exploring the qualities of one flower. Then, when your mind grows restless, shift your focus to the flower in the next corner, and so on. You should visualize each clearly.

Tratak

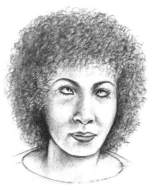

Tratak or steady gazing is an excellent concentration exercise. It involves alternately gazing at an object or point without blinking, then closing your eyes and visualizing the object in your mind's eye. The practice steadies the wandering mind and concentrates the attention, leading you to focus with pin-point accuracy. Wherever the eyes go, the mind follows, so that when you fix your gaze on a single point, the mind too becomes one-pointed. Though primarily intended to strengthen your powers of concentration and purify the mind, Tratak also improves the eyesight and stimulates the brain via the optic nerve. It is one of the six purification practices called Kriyas.

Tratak is most commonly performed with a candle (as described on p.96) but you can equally well use various other objects as targets for your gaze. You can mark a black dot on a piece of paper and attach it to the wall or use a chakra (p.71) or a yantra (p.96). Yantras are geometrical diagrams which serve to focus the mind. Like a mantra, each yantra has a specific mystical meaning. Alternatively, you can try gazing at a symbol, such as OM (p.96), or at the image of a deity. There is no need to restrict your practice to objects indoors – the natural world offers a wealth of suitable focusing points. In the daytime, a flower or a shell can act as a target of attention, while at night you might try fixing your gaze on the moon or a bright star. So long as your object of concentration is unmoving and relatively small to the gaze, focusing on it will produce the desired effect. Yogis often use the space between the eyebrows or the tip of the nose for Tratak, as shown above

The technique of Tratak remains much the same, whatever the target of your gaze is, though naturally you will have to adapt it slightly when meditating out of doors. Place your chosen object at eye level, about three feet away from you. First regulate your breathing, then start to gaze at the object without blinking. Don't stare or gaze vacantly – just look steadily, without straining. After about a minute, close your eyes and, keeping your inner gaze steady, visualize the object at the Ajna or Anahata chakra (see p.92). When the after-image vanishes, open your eyes again and repeat. The Hatha Yoga Pradipika directs: "Look with fixed eyes at a minute object with concentration till tears are shed". If your eyes do indeed water after gazing for a short while, it is simply a sign to close them – you will gradually be able to extend the period of gazing. As your concentration grows deeper and your gaze steadier, lengthen the times spent with eyes open then closed until you are practising for up to an hour. In your early days of Tratak, you may find unwanted thoughts intruding on your mind. Just keep bringing your attention back to the object of concentration and your mind will become more focused. With practice you will be able to visualize your chosen object quite clearly when you close your eyes.

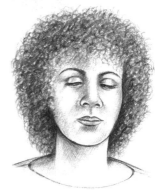

Frontal and Nasal Gazing
Gazing at the point between your eyebrows, seat of the "third eye" (top) or at the tip of your nose (below) strengthens your eye muscles, besides improving your concentration. One minute of gazing is sufficient to start with, building up to ten minutes. Don't strain the eyes – if they feel sore or tired, close them at once. Frontal Gazing awakens Kundalini, while Nasal Gazing affects the central nervous system.

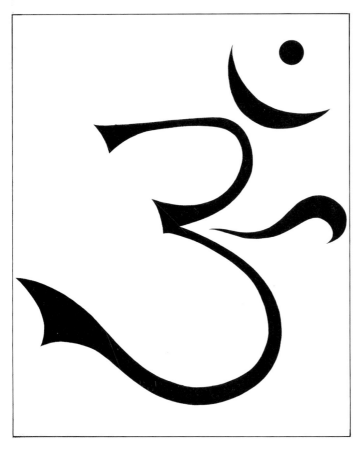

OM

To a yogi, no symbol is more powerful than the syllable OM, as witnessed by these words from the Mandukya Up-anishad: "OM: this eternal word is all; what was, what is and what shall be." In the Sanskrit letter the long lower curve represents the dream state, the upper curve stands for the waking state and the curve issuing from the centre symbolizes deep, dreamless sleep. The crescent shape stands for "maya", the veil of illusion and the dot for the transcendental state. When the individual spirit in man passes through the veil and rests in the transcendental he is liberated from the three states and their qualities.

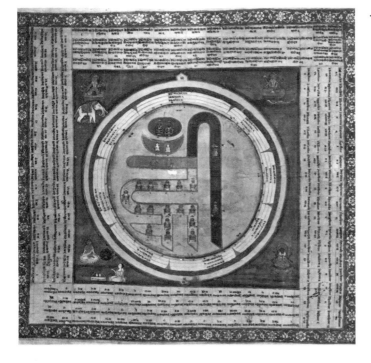

Tratak on OM
When using the Sanskrit OM (top left) for tratak, let your eyes walk over it in an anti-clockwise direction. In the 18th-century OM Yantra (below left) the sacred syllable is represented in a different form. The yantra originates from Rajasthan in India.

Candle Gazing *(right)*
A candle flame is the most widely used object for tratak, as it is easy to hold an after-image of the bright flame when you close your eyes. You should place the candle at eye level in a darkened, draught-free room.

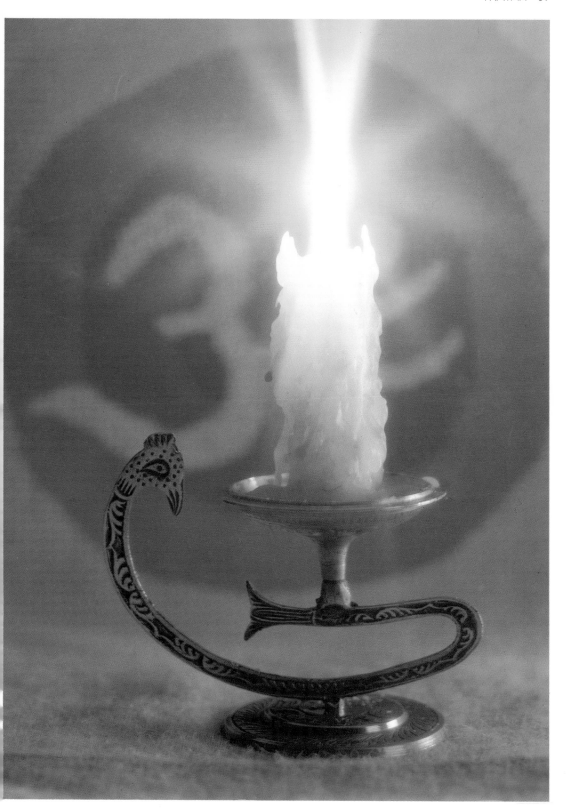

Mantras

Sound is a form of energy made up of vibrations or wavelengths – certain wavelengths have the power to heal, others are capable of shattering glass. Mantras are Sanskrit syllables, words or phrases which, when repeated in meditation, will bring the individual to a higher state of consciousness. They are sounds or energies that have always existed in the universe and can neither be created nor destroyed. There are six qualities common to any true mantra: it was originally revealed to and handed on by a sage who attained self-realization through it; it has a certain metre and a presiding deity; it has a "bija" or seed at its essence which invests it with special power; it has divine cosmic energy or shakti; and lastly it has a key which must be unlocked through constant repetition before pure consciousness is revealed. Japa or mantra repetition not only provides you with a tangible point on which to focus your mind – it also releases the energy encased in that sound. The energy literally manifests itself, creating a specific thought pattern in the mind. Correct pronunciation is therefore very important. With sincere practice, repetition of a mantra leads to pure thought where the sound vibration merges with the thought vibration and there is no awareness of meaning. In this way the mantra will lead you to true meditation, to a state of oneness, of non-duality. There are three main types of mantra: Saguna mantras invoke specific deities or aspects of the Absolute; Nirguna mantras are abstract and declare the meditator's identification with the Absolute; and "Bija" or seed mantras are aspects of OM and derive directly from the fifty primeval sounds. It is best to be initiated into a mantra by a guru, who will invest it with his own pranic energy. But if this is not possible, practise repeating the mantras and choose one that feels comfortable. Bija mantras are not included, since they are too powerful to be used by beginners.

Forms of japa

You can repeat your mantra out loud – by saying or chanting it – in a whisper, or mentally. Mental japa is the most effective, because mantras are on a wavelength far beyond "voiced" or physical sound. But at the beginning, when keeping the mind focused is more of a problem, you should start your meditation by voicing the mantra, then whisper it, before turning to mental repetition. Whichever form of japa you use, it is helpful to coordinate the mantra with your breathing. In addition three techniques of japa will aid your powers of concentration. You can use a string of beads called a "mala" (shown to the right), repeating your mantra as you count along the beads. You can use the thumb of your right hand as a pointer to count along the lines between your finger joints, as shown top right. And lastly, you can write the mantra down at the same time as repeating it mentally (see opposite).

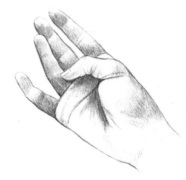

Finger-line counting
Place your right thumb on the top line of your little finger and move it on each time you repeat the mantra – first to the middle line, then the lowest line, then on to the lines of the fourth finger, and so on. Using the three lines of the four fingers is twelve repetitions; nine rounds adds up to a hundred and eight repetitions, or one mala.

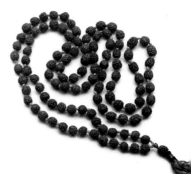

Using a mala
A mala has one hundred and eight beads plus the larger "meru" bead. Holding it in the right hand, start at the meru and roll the beads along one by one between your thumb and third fingers while repeating your mantra. When you reach the meru, roll the mala in the opposite direction. Don't cross over the meru bead.

Saguna Mantras

राम्

Ram (rahm)
The energy pattern for truth, righteousness and virtue in their male aspect, this powerful mantra is made up of three seed sounds.

सीता

Sita (see-tah)
This is the female aspect of the energy pattern of Ram. It stands for the descent of Prakriti or nature (p.16) in the form of the mother. It can also be repeated with Ram as Sitaram : when joined together the two mantras embody the energy existing in an ideal marriage or union.

श्याम्

Shyam (shyahm)
Representing cosmic love and compassion in the male aspect, this mantra transmutes all emotions into unconditional love.

राधा

Radha (rah-duh)
Radha is the female aspect of Shyam, symbolizing the cosmic love of the divine mother.

ॐ नमः शिवाय

Om Namah Sivaya (ohm nuh-muh shivai-uh)
This is a purifying energy pattern that destroys our negative qualities, chosen especially by those of an ascetic nature. The dance of Siva represents the movement inherent in matter. When Siva stops dancing, the illusion of matter is destroyed.

ॐ नमो नारायणाय

Om Namo Narayanaya (ohm nuh-mo nah-rai-uh-nai-uh)
The energy pattern of harmony and balance in their male aspect, this mantra is used especially by people in times of trouble, to bring them the strength to regain harmony in their lives.

ॐ ऐं सरस्वतै नमः

Om Aim Saraswatyai Namah (ohm aym suh-ruh-swht-yai nuh-muh-huh)
The female aspect of the pattern of creative energy and wisdom, this mantra is often chosen by artists and musicians.

Nirguna Mantras

ॐ

Om (ohm)
Om is the original mantra, the root of all sounds and letters, and thus of all language and thought. The "O" is generated deep within the body, and slowly brought upward joining with the "m" which then resonates through the entire head. Repeating Om for twenty minutes relaxes every atom in your body.

सोऽहम्

Soham (soh-hum)
This mantra is unconsciously repeated each time we take a breath – inhaling "So", exhaling "ham". It means "I am That" – beyond the limitations of mind and body, at one with the Absolute.

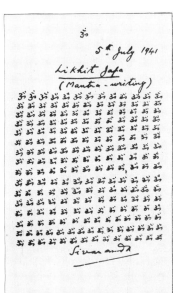

Likhita Japa
If you want to do Likhita japa or mantra writing, you should set aside a special notebook for the purpose. Before you start, decide how many times you will repeat the mantra or for how long. The aim is not to write as quickly as possible, but to give due consideration to every single repetition. You can either use Sanskrit or the transliterated version to write your chosen mantra. Instead of just working from left to right, try making patterns with your mantra writing too. Shown above is an example of Swami Sivananda's own Likhita Japa.

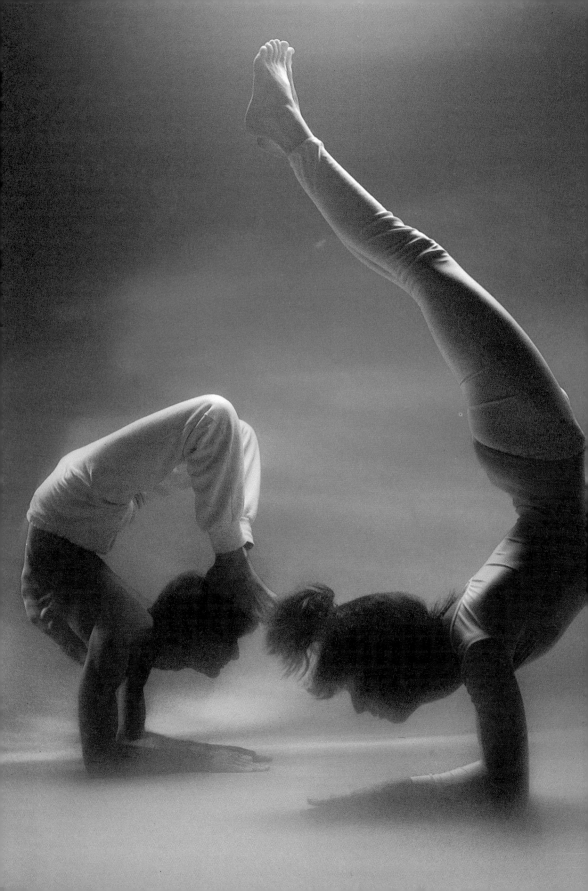

Asanas and Variations

"The posture becomes perfect,
when the effort of achieving
it vanishes."
Yogabhashya

In the Basic Session, you learned the blue-print for your daily practice. This chapter expands your scope, presenting a wide range of variations and new asanas for you to incorporate into this pattern. For the sake of clarity we have divided the asanas into six cycles – the Headstand Cycle, the Shoulderstand Cycle, the Forward Bend Cycle, the Backward Bend Cycle, the Sitting Cycle and the Balancing Cycle. These cycles are not designed to create rigid divisions between postures, but rather to show where each asana belongs in the scheme of things.

Every cycle contains variations of asanas from the Basic Session, plus new asanas that belong to the same family group. In general each double-page spread is organized so that the easier asanas come first and the more advanced ones last. Often the more advanced variations are simply natural progressions of the easier ones, which you will come to in time as your strength and flexibility develop. But however adept you are, you should proceed systematically rather than skipping about at random, to warm up your body for the more difficult poses.

Don't expect to practise the whole of each cycle in one go. Select a few new asanas or variations from every cycle and incorporate them in your basic session, which by now should be second nature to you. Take care to divide your time fairly evenly between the cycles – it is essential that you keep a balance if you are not to strengthen one aspect of your asanas at the expense of another. Similarly, get in the habit of balancing the variations you perform – counter a forward-bending variation, for example, with a backward-bending one. Always go gently when learning new asanas especially if you are relatively stiff to begin with. This is not only to avoid over-stretching your muscles or joints, but also to accustom your internal organs to being moved, in unfamiliar ways.

You may find that you make quite rapid progress to begin with, but then appear to reach a plateau where you notice no improvement. Don't be despondent if this happens – you are making progress, even if you are not aware of it. Continue your daily practice as usual, trying different variations to keep your mind stimulated, and you will soon pass this stretch. In time you will gain a wider perspective of the part asanas play in your everyday life and cease to rely on the "kick" of becoming more advanced.

For some yogis, one pose suffices to reach perfection – they will hold a Headstand, say, for three hours at a time. But most people need to evolve more gradually, working through a variety of movements. Different asanas affect different areas of the body and mind. As various parts of the body open up and come under your control, there is often a corresponding "opening up" of the personality, as well as a heightened awareness. This can manifest itself in a variety of ways, both emotionally and spiritually – you may discover that you feel more open and relaxed in company, for example, and that meditation comes more easily. It is while you hold an asana that your body really begins to open up. Close your eyes and use the time to concentrate on your breathing or repeat a mantra. Performing the variations of one of the basic asanas, such as the Shoulderstand, strengthens your control in that asana and enables you to hold it steadily. The steadier you can hold a pose, the freer your mind is to turn inward in meditation.

The Headstand Cycle

Once you have mastered the basic Headstand and grown accustomed to being upside-down, you can begin to explore the space around your inverted body, to add movement and depth to the central pose. In fact, all the variations in this cycle are perfectly natural outgrowths of the Headstand – left to your own devices, you would intuitively find them by yourself. One of the main lessons you are learning in the inverted poses is to regard your arms and legs as interchangeable. With practice, your arms will carry your weight as easily as your legs do, allowing you the same range of movements when inverted that you enjoy when standing up. The Headstand is by nature a very meditative pose. Take advantage of this fact while you hold the variations – let the mind become still and one pointed.

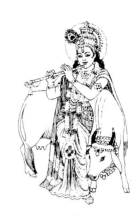

Leg Raising Variations

You must be able to support your own weight without strain if you are to enjoy the more advanced asanas and be able to meditate in them. The leg-raising movements shown here are a means to this higher goal. By learning to support the weight of your legs from a supine position you will develop the strength you need to support and control the entire weight of your body in other poses. In time you can replace these exercises with leg-lifting variations in standing or inverted asanas. In Variation 1, you use your legs like "weights", swinging them in an arc from one side to the other. Variation 2 stretches your legs and gives increased mobility in the hip joints. Try to repeat each exercise at least three times, making sure that your shoulders remain on the floor and that your knees are straight.

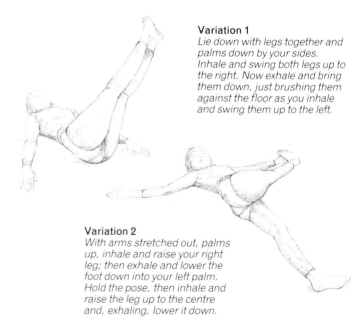

Variation 1
Lie down with legs together and palms down by your sides. Inhale and swing both legs up to the right. Now exhale and bring them down, just brushing them against the floor as you inhale and swing them up to the left.

Variation 2
With arms stretched out, palms up, inhale and raise your right leg; then exhale and lower the foot down into your left palm. Hold the pose, then inhale and raise the leg up to the centre and, exhaling, lower it down.

Headstand Leg Variations

To perform any of the variations shown right and opposite you should be confident of your Sirshasana. Keep both legs straight in the poses, holding them for as long as they are comfortable. Once these leg movements become effortless, you can dispense with the leg raises from the floor.

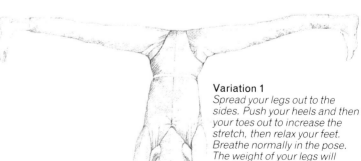

Variation 1
Spread your legs out to the sides. Push your heels and then your toes out to increase the stretch, then relax your feet. Breathe normally in the pose. The weight of your legs will gradually pull them wider apart.

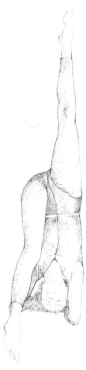

Variations 2 and 3
2 *Pulling your hips back, exhale and lower one leg to the floor without transferring any weight to the foot. Inhale; raise the leg.*
3 *(right) From Variation 1, exhale and lower one leg down by your side. Inhaling, raise it.*

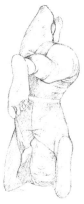

Variation 4
Move your right leg straight forward and your left leg back. Point your heels, then point your toes. Let gravity pull your legs down further. Now bring your legs back to the Headstand and repeat, reversing the legs.

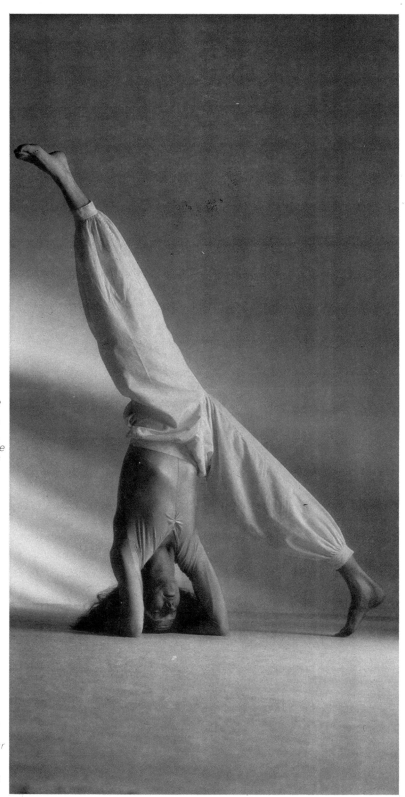

The Scorpion

Mastering Vrischikasana, the Scorpion, is more a matter of confidence and concentration than of strength. Think of your hands and forearms as giant "feet" and you will soon overcome any fears of falling. In fact, when resting on hands and forearms your weight is distributed over a much larger area than when standing up. Before you attempt the full Scorpion, get used to arching your body backward, unclasping your fingers and changing hand positions, then clasping your hands again and coming back into the Headstand. When learning the asana, try to bring your chest and legs as near to the floor as you can and pull your hips backward, away from your feet, to steady yourself. Success in holding the pose lies mainly in bringing your legs over far enough to offset the weight of your torso, and in using your hands to keep your balance. After you practise the Scorpion, counterstretch the spine by performing a forward bend in the Headstand, bringing your feet down in front of your face to the floor (p. 103).

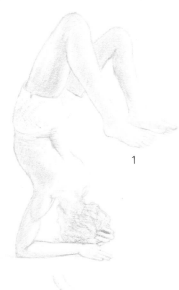

1

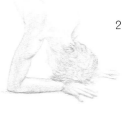

2

1 Arch your back and, bending your knees, separate your legs and bring them down behind you. Unclasp your fingers and place one hand flat on the floor by your head.
2 Place the other hand flat, then move your wrists out slightly so that your hands and forearms are parallel. Push your shoulders up to the ceiling, taking all the weight off your head.

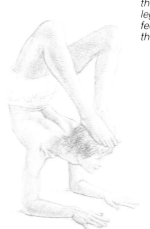

3 Now lift up your head and hold the pose. With practice, your legs will drop down so that your feet touch your head. Reverse the steps to come down.

Variation 1
When you become more adept, try straightening your legs from the classic position. Once you have mastered this you can come directly into the straight-legged Scorpion without bending your legs first.

Variation 2
It is in this advanced variation (shown far right) that the pose most resembles a scorpion with its tail arched over its back. Bring your legs over as low to the floor as possible. Pull your hips back as far as you can and try to straighten your knees.

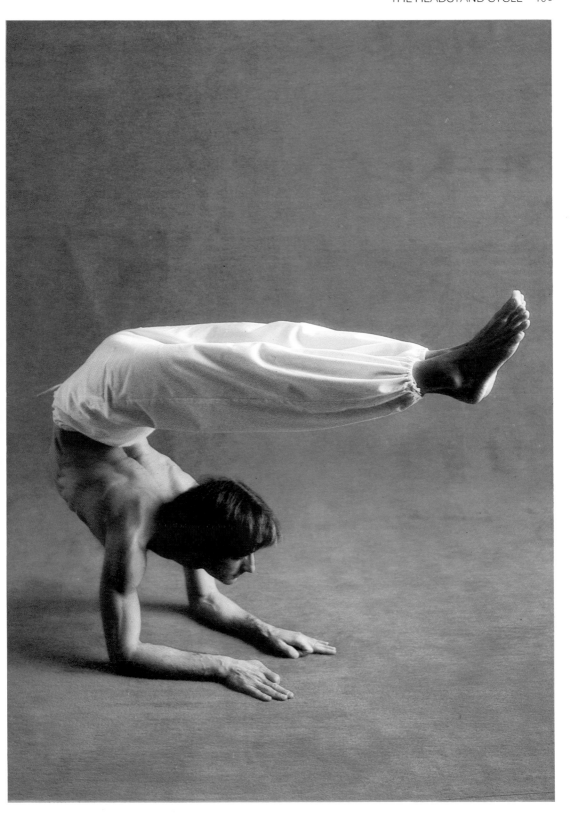

Arm Variations

Once you are sure of your Headstand, try replacing its "tripod"
base with alternative arm positions. Moving into and holding
these arm variations is a lesson
in balance. If you find it too hard
to move your arms with your
legs in the classic Sirshasana
(as shown), open your legs out
to the sides (p. 102) – the nearer
your body is to the floor, the
easier it is to balance. As you
shift your weight to alter the
position of your arms, keep your
mind steady by controlling your
breathing. Each time you meet
and overcome a new obstacle in
your asanas, you will gain confidence in your ability to transcend your own limitations.

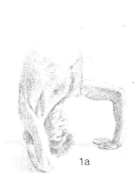

1a

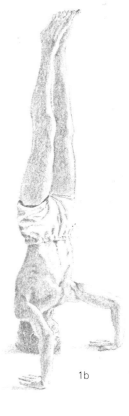

1a *Unclasp your hands and
transfer most of your weight to
your left side. When you feel
balanced, inhale and, retaining
your breath, bring your right
hand back and place it where
the elbow was.*
1b *Now repeat on the other side,
bringing your left hand back.
Hold, breathing normally.*

1b

2a

2b

2a *Transfer your weight to your
left side again, inhale and, as
you retain the breath, stretch
your right arm out straight in
front of you, palm down.*
2b *Repeat on the other side,
stretching the left arm out. Your
arms should be shoulder-width
apart. Hold, breathing normally.
In an even more advanced variation, you move your arms
straight out in front with elbows
and forearms touching,(far right).*

3a *Once again, shift your weight
to your left side. Inhale, and as
you retain the breath, bend your
right arm and place the forearm
down in front of your face.*
3b *Repeat, bringing the left arm
in over the right and wrapping
your hands round your arms.
Hold, then come down — or
reverse the steps to come down
from the classic Headstand.*

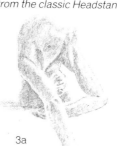

3a

3b

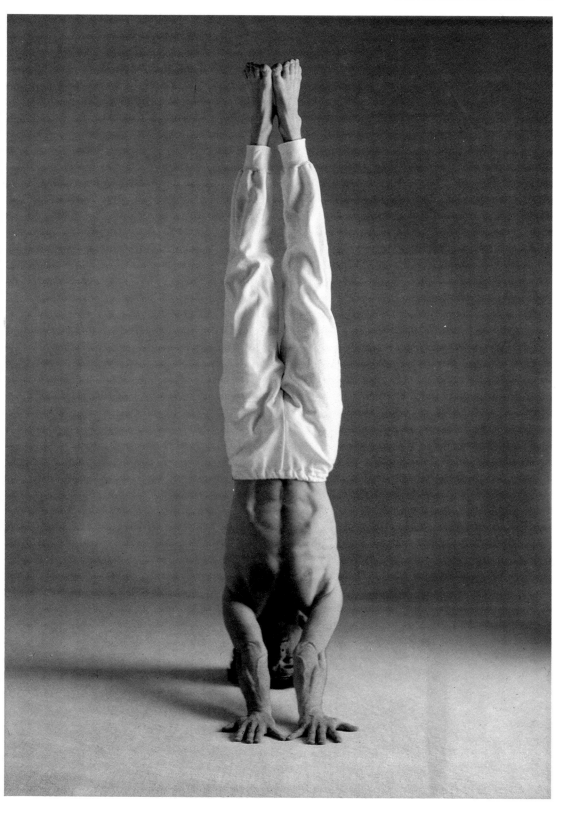

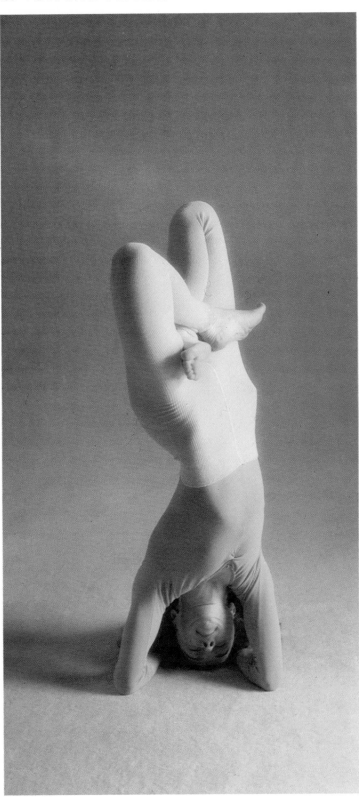

The Lotus Headstand

When you practise the Lotus Headstand (Oordhwapadmasana), you are making your inverted body more compact. With your legs securely folded it is in fact easier to support your weight and hold steady in the Headstand. Locking your limbs also helps to free you from the distractions of the body, allowing you to turn your attention inward. The Headstand draws prana down to the brain, the Lotus contains it in the lower limbs. When you combine the two asanas, you can feel the pranic energy centred in your spine. In addition to the twist, shown left, you can also fold forward in the pose. With your legs in the Lotus there is less strain on your lower back, giving you a more thorough bend.

The Lotus Headstand
Come into the Lotus in the Headstand. After bringing one leg in, bend your hips forward a little, to help position the second leg.

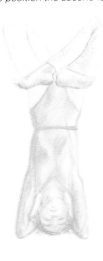

Variation *(left)*
Twist your hips to the right while pushing down on your left forearm to help balance yourself. Repeat, twisting to the left.

Single Leg Inverted Pose

This is one of the most advanced positions of the Headstand Cycle, demanding great flexibility and strength. Arching the spine right back you bring your feet to the floor behind your head, then raise one leg at a time, giving a powerful stretch to each side of your body in turn. The pose also strengthens the legs and feet, for in addition to bearing the body's weight the foot that remains on the floor provides leverage for your hands to pull your upper spine and head backward. When you perform this asana, concentrate on lifting your head up toward your standing leg.

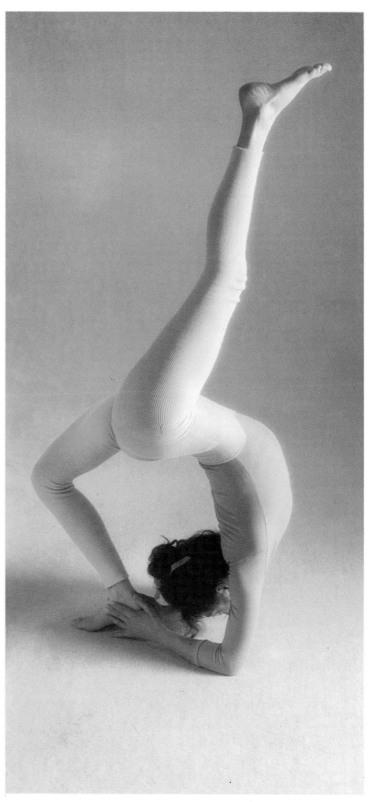

1 *In the Headstand, arch your back and bring your legs over behind your head. Then press your elbows firmly against the floor, relax your back, and push your hips up as you gently drop down on your feet. (If you are unready to drop over from the Headstand, push up into this position from the floor, with your arms in the Headstand "tripod".)*

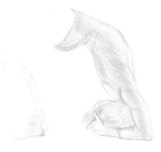

2 *Now unclasp your fingers and walk one foot back toward your head. Holding the foot in both hands, lift the other leg straight up, as shown right, and raise your head off the floor. Repeat, raising the opposite leg.*

The Shoulderstand Cycle

The asanas in this cycle are mentally far more approachable than those in the Headstand Cycle, for the simple reason that with your head face up on the floor, you can see what you are doing. This not only reduces your fear of pitching your body into new positions, but also means that you can act as your own teacher, checking that your body is straight or your limbs are symmetrical. The cycle concentrates prana on the neck and upper spine area and this in turn brings great benefit to the lower back – since any work done at one end of the spine is automatically reflected at the other end. In order to come into these variations correctly, pull your shoulders down and stretch your neck up, away from the shoulders, while you are still lying in the Corpse Pose (pp. 24-25).

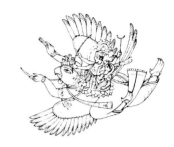

Arm Variations

The more adept you become at asanas, the less you need to use your arms to support your body – you will soon find, for example, that you can stand up from sitting on the floor without the aid of your hands. To balance in Sarvangasana with your arms inverted by your sides (as in Variation 3), you must have strong back muscles and good concentration. Once you can do it, try practising Leg Variations with your arms up too.

Leg Variations

One of the chief lessons of the inverted poses is to teach you to regard your legs as "balancers" as well as weight-bearing objects. In both the Shoulderstand and Headstand, the Leg Variations change your perception of balance and alter the way your weight is distributed.

Variation 1
With your back supported, exhale as you lower your right leg to the floor behind your head. Inhale and bring it back up. Keep both legs straight. Repeat three times with each leg.

Variation 3
Come into the Shoulderstand, supporting your back in the normal way. Now slowly bring first your right, then your left arm, up alongside your hips. Hold the position, breathing normally.
Note *You should only practise this arm variation if you can keep your back straight – if your body sags down when you move your arms up, support your back.*

Variation 2
Lower the right leg, as in Variation 1. Stretch your left arm out along the floor behind your back, bend your leg and bring the knee down by your ear. Clasp your foot in your right hand. Repeat with the left leg.

Variation 4
With your back supported, bend your right knee slightly, then cross your left leg over it and wrap your left foot around your right ankle. Squeeze your legs together. After holding the pose, repeat with the right leg wrapped around the left. This is the Eagle Shoulderstand.

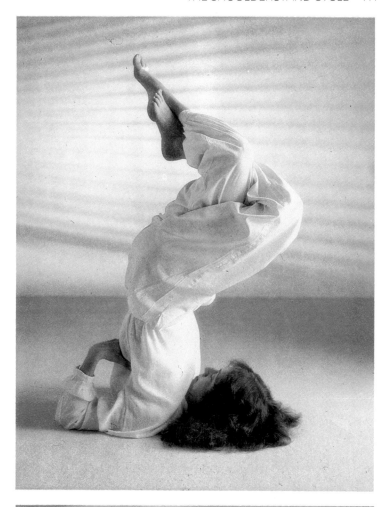

Variation 5
With your back supported in the Shoulderstand, bend your right knee and place the foot on the left thigh in the Half Lotus. Inhale. Now exhale and lower your left foot to the floor behind your head. Inhale and raise it. Repeat, changing legs.

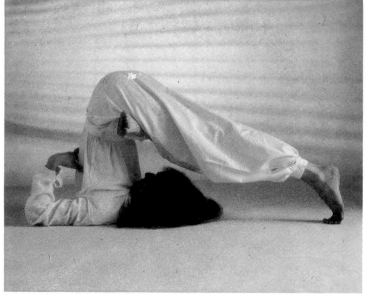

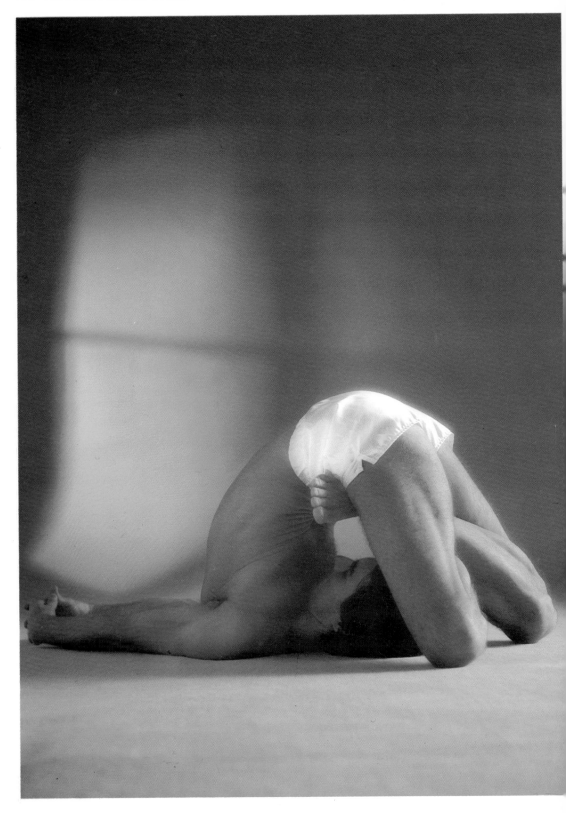

Plough Variations

The variations of the Plough (Halasana) bend and stretch each part of your spine in turn. With legs stretched out away from your head you are working on your neck and upper spine, while walking your feet in close to your head moves the stretch down to your lower back. Before practising any of these variations, always hold the classic pose, with hands clasped behind your back. Whenever you feel stiff in a position at first, bring your arms over to the floor behind you for a short time, to relieve the stretch on your upper back. If you find yourself resorting to fast, shallow breathing in these variations, relax into the pose and focus your mind on your breath. This will soon overcome the problem.

Ear to Knee

In the Plough, exhale, bend your legs and lower your knees to the floor by your ears. Wrap your arms over your knees and press your palms over your ears.
Variation 1 *With straight legs, walk your feet as far apart as possible. Stretch your arms straight up between your legs, with your hands in the prayer position. In this pose your spine, rather than your shoulders, is carrying all your weight.*

Variations 2 and 3

2a *Interlock your fingers behind your back. Now walk your feet as far as possible to one side, keeping your knees straight and your legs as shown left.*
2b *Exhale, bend your knees and bring them down by your ear. Repeat both these steps on the other side.*

2 *(below) Walk your feet as far back from your head as possible. Exhale, bend your knees and bring them down to the floor. Pressing your arms and*

3 *(below) Walk your feet as far back from your head as possible. Exhale, bend your knees and bring them down to the floor. Pressing your arms and*

Variation 4 *(left)*
Come into the Shoulderstand and bring your legs into the Lotus. Slowly lower your knees to the floor behind your head.

Bridge Variations

Practising Sethu Bandhasana and its variations develops tremendous strength in the lower back and abdomen. By holding the hips up high you are resisting the pull of gravity. In Variation 1 the pose is a little easier to maintain, as the raised leg helps you to keep the body up. Once you have no difficulty coming down into the Bridge from the Shoulderstand with both legs at once, move your hands down nearer your shoulderblades. Make sure your elbows don't bow outward when you come into the pose. Whenever an asana or variation becomes effortless, look for ways of perfecting it. Don't become complacent. No matter how adept you are there is always one more step you can take. In the case of the Bridge, for instance, you might perhaps try coming out of the Shoulderstand with one leg in the Half Lotus and one leg straight.

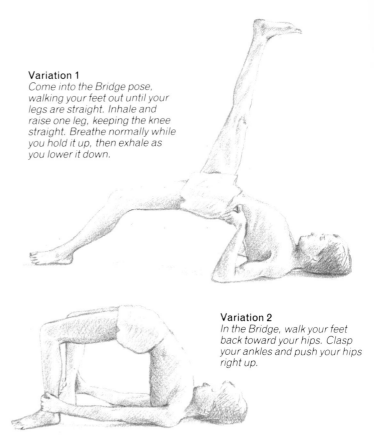

Variation 1
Come into the Bridge pose, walking your feet out until your legs are straight. Inhale and raise one leg, keeping the knee straight. Breathe normally while you hold it up, then exhale as you lower it down.

Variation 2
In the Bridge, walk your feet back toward your hips. Clasp your ankles and push your hips right up.

Variation 3 *(right)*
Come into the lotus pose in the Shoulderstand. Supporting your back firmly, exhale and slowly lower your knees. Keep your head and shoulders down and your elbows in position.

Fish Variations

Yogis use the Lotus Fish to float in water for long periods, combining the pose with a special breathing technique. When your spine is arched back in these Matsyasana variations, prana is directed upward to the chest and head – locking your legs in the Lotus pose prevents loss of prana through the lower limbs. To increase the arch in your back and open up the chest area to expand the lungs, lever yourself up further by pulling on your feet and pressing down with your elbows. Try to get the crown of your head on the floor so that you can feel the bend extending to your upper spine.

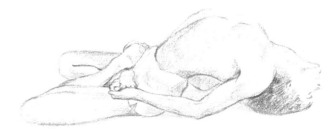

Variation 1 (Lotus Fish)
Lie down with your legs in the Lotus. Leaning on your elbows, arch your back up until you are resting on the top of your head. Hold your feet from below, palms up, and try to press your elbows to the floor and your knees down.

Variation 2 (Bound Fish)
In the Lotus Fish, transfer your weight to your left elbow, keeping your back arched, as shown right. Reach under your back with the right arm. Inhale and clasp the right foot. Exhale. Now repeat with the other arm.

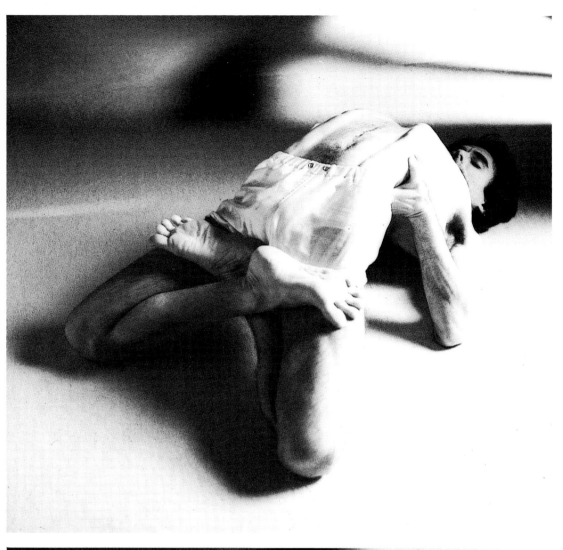

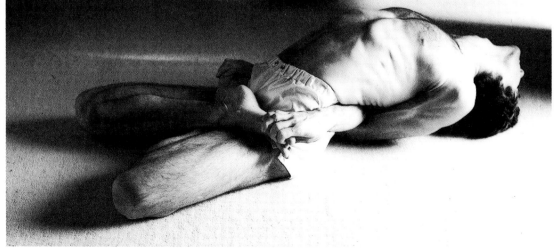

The Forward Bend Cycle

This cycle encompasses not only the forward-bending asanas and variations, but also their counterpose – the Inclined Plane. The forward bends stretch and lengthen the natural curve of your spine, creating space between the vertebrae. With time and repeated practice, this stretching exercise educates the back muscles to keep the vertebrae properly aligned. It also enables the spine to bend further back in the opposite direction – thus, as you progress with the asanas in this cycle, your backward bends will improve. If you squeeze part of your body – your arm, for example – it goes red because more blood is brought to the area. The forward bends squeeze the abdominal organs, nourishing them with fresh blood, and thus keeping the entire digestive system healthy. The cycle as a whole also has a beneficial effect on the mind.

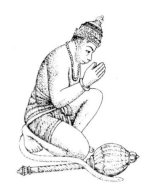

Forward Bend Variations

The key to mastering this series lies in learning how to extend forward right from the base of your spine, while keeping the backs of your knees on the floor. The various handholds alter the pull on your spine and shoulders – and offer different methods of levering yourself further into the pose. Variation 5 demands a good sense of balance as well as strength, while Variation 6 gives the torso a powerful stretch and tones the abdominal organs. Try to hold all these Paschimothanasana variations for a long time, readjusting the body to increase the stretch. You can elongate the spine a great deal — In time, you may succeed in touching your feet with your head.

Variations 1 and 2
1 *Wrap your palms around your soles, fingers under your heels. This variation increases the stretch on your hamstrings.*
2 *(below) With your elbows on the floor, interlock your fingers around your arches.*

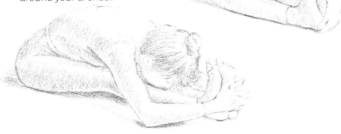

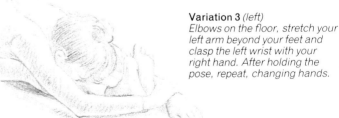

Variation 3 *(left)*
Elbows on the floor, stretch your left arm beyond your feet and clasp the left wrist with your right hand. After holding the pose, repeat, changing hands.

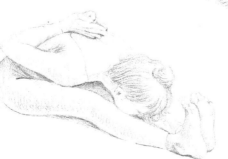

Variation 4
Sit up straight with your legs together in front of you. Join your palms behind your back. Now stretch forward from the base of the spine, using the muscles of your abdomen and back. This pose opens up the shoulders and allows you to press the spine down gently with your joined hands.

Variation 5

Sit down with your knees bent in to your chest. Hold your toes and lean back a little way, balancing on your buttocks. Slowly straighten your legs, bringing your thighs to your chest and drawing your head and spine up toward your feet. To develop your abdominal muscles, try raising your legs with your hands – palms down – by your sides.

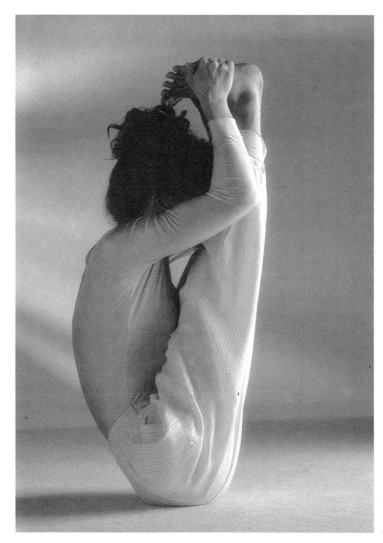

Variation 6

In the Forward Bend, twist your body to the right, bringing your left elbow down to the floor beside your right shin. Use the elbow to lever your torso into the twist. Now hold the right foot with your left hand and raise your right hand over your head to hold the left foot. Look up between your elbows. Hold the position, breathing normally; then repeat, twisting to the left.

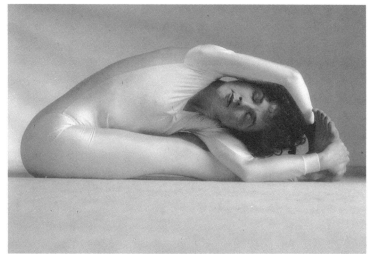

The Head to Knee Pose

In Janu Sirasana, the bent leg gives support and leverage while the straight leg is stretched by the weight of the torso, loosening the hamstrings. You will find that you can bend further down over one leg than over two, as it is easier to stretch one side at a time. This series of asanas has a powerful effect on the abdominal organs. The massage they receive in Janu Sirasana itself (centre right) is intensified by performing the pose in the Half Lotus. The twisting movements of Variations 2 and 3 reach deep inside, purifying the system and making the whole body lean. Start each asana by bending over the right leg, to tone the ascending colon; then repeat on the left, to tone the descending colon. In Variation 2, try to push out your chest. Once you can perform the pose without effort, progress to Variation 3.

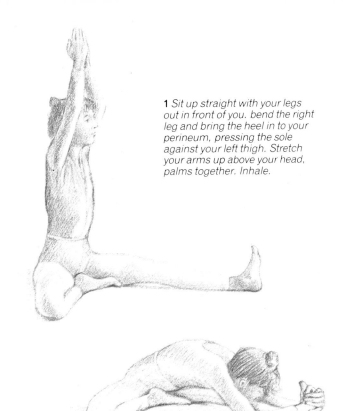

1 Sit up straight with your legs out in front of you. bend the right leg and bring the heel in to your perineum, pressing the sole against your left thigh. Stretch your arms up above your head, palms together. Inhale.

2 (above) Exhale and fold forward from the base of your spine. Clasping your foot in both hands, bring your head down your leg as far as possible. Breathe deeply in the position; then release it slowly.

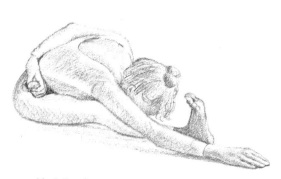

Variation 1
Place your left foot in the Half Lotus. Reach behind your back with your left hand and hold the foot. Inhale. Now exhale and bend forward over your right leg. If this is too advanced, fold forward without holding the foot.

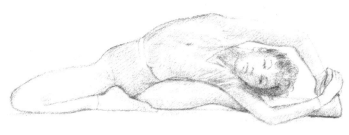

Variations 2 and 3
2 (above) Push your knee back in line with the left foot. Exhale; bend left. Holding the foot, use the left elbow to lever the right arm back.
3 (right) Release the left hand; move shoulder out to bring head to floor. Now roll the head back on to the leg, face up, and clasp the foot.

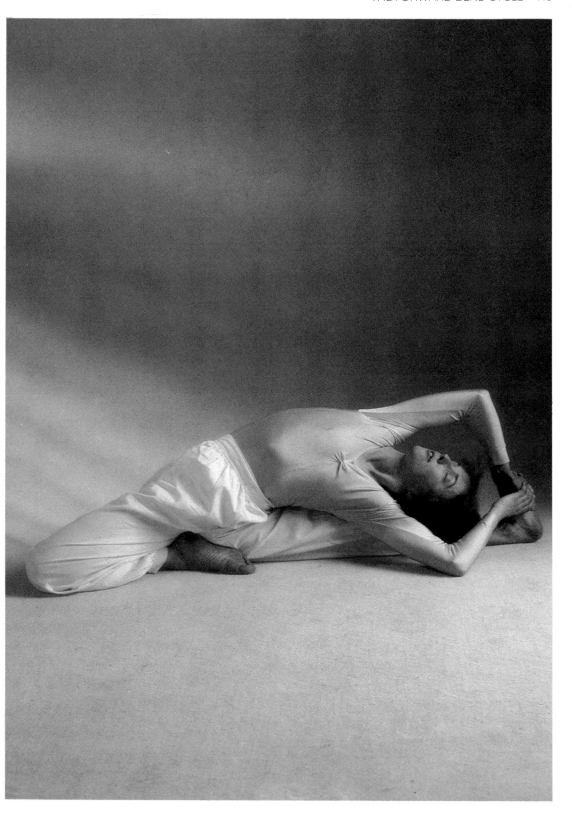

The Side Splits Twists

A good stretch is like a yawn – if you don't complete it you feel unsatisfied. Keep stretching your legs apart gently and in time they will gradually open up into the Side Splits. Start both these twisting asanas by spreading your legs as far apart as comfort permits, rotating them backward from the hips – the wider you stretch them, the easier it will be to twist sideways. Try to lengthen your spine as you bend to the side, to bring your head right down to your foot. Once in position, pull your toes back toward your head, then push your heels out, to increase the stretch and help you to balance.

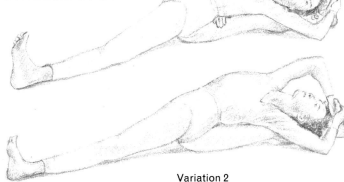

Variation 1
Reach behind your back with your right hand and hold your inner left thigh. Exhale and lay your torso on your left leg. Clasp the foot in your left hand.

Variation 2
From Variation 1, release the right hand to hold the left foot. Move the left elbow and shoulder out from the leg. Now lay your head on your shin.

Leg and Arm Stretching

In these two Hastha Padasana variations, your legs are slightly rotated and stretched by the weight of your body as you bend forward. Gravity assists you by pulling your body down. Take care to avoid overstretching your legs by taking most of your weight on your hands at first. Little by little inch your way forward until you can bring your elbows down. By the time you can rest your chin and chest on the floor, your inner thighs will have stretched sufficiently.

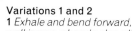

Variations 1 and 2
1 Exhale and bend forward, walking your hands along the floor until both legs and spine reach their maximum stretch.
2 Stretch your legs out and clasp your toes. Now bend forward, leading with the chest, spreading your legs apart.

The Tortoise
For Kurmasana, sit with your legs apart, knees up and feet flat on the floor. Bend forward and bring your arms and shoulders under your knees, hands pointing backward, palms down. Slowly stretch your legs out, pull your torso forward.

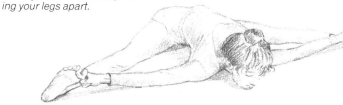

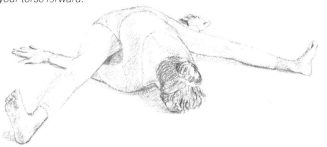

The Balancing Tortoise *(right)*
For Uthitha Kurmasana, inhale, then exhale, raise your right leg and bring it behind your head. Repeat, bringing the left leg up and behind the right, locking the ankles. Breathe normally in the pose. On an inhalation, lift your body and balance on your hands.

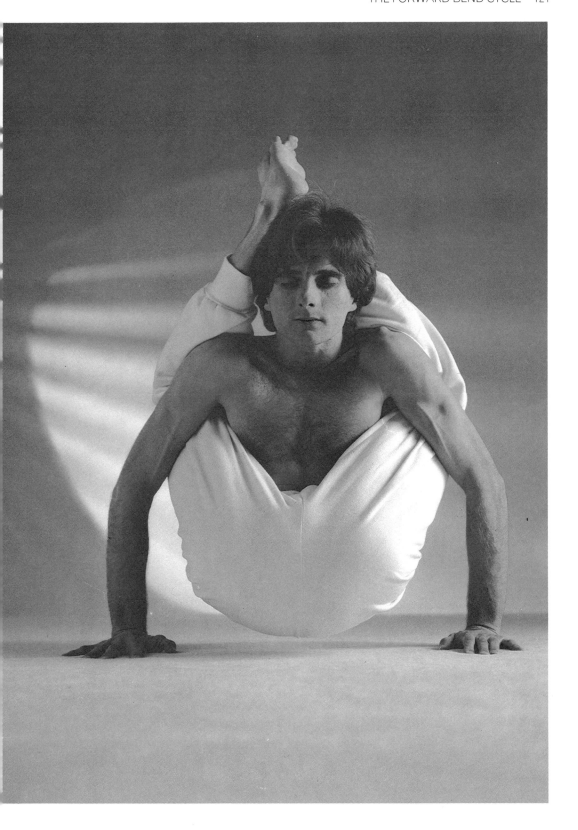

The Inclined Plane

This asana is a counterpose to the forward bends, just as the Fish complements the other asanas in the Shoulderstand Cycle. Having brought your head and spine forward over your legs, you now tilt the body up and drop your head back. This stretches the entire front of your body from the top of your head to your toes. The higher you push your hips, the more you will increase the stretch and strengthen your legs, shoulders and arms. Once you can bring your hips up far enough, your spine and back muscles will share in supporting your body. Practising the variations strengthens all parts of the body in turn and heightens your awareness of any imbalances between your left and right sides. At first you may find it uncomfortable to hold these positions, or hard to balance in them – keep repeating them, then relaxing, and in the course of time you will build up enough strength to perform the complete sequence.

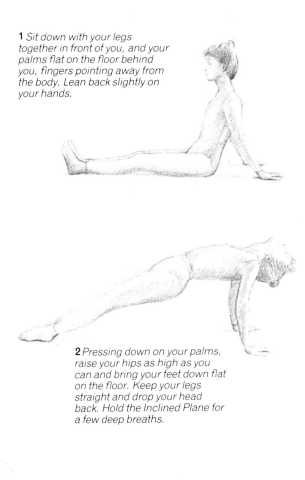

1 *Sit down with your legs together in front of you, and your palms flat on the floor behind you, fingers pointing away from the body. Lean back slightly on your hands.*

2 *Pressing down on your palms, raise your hips as high as you can and bring your feet down flat on the floor. Keep your legs straight and drop your head back. Hold the Inclined Plane for a few deep breaths.*

Variation 1
From the Inclined Plane, inhale and raise the right leg straight up, keeping the left foot flat on the floor. Hold the position, breathing deeply, then release it and repeat, raising the left leg.

Variation 2
From the Inclined Plane, inhale and raise your right arm – you need to lean slightly to the left. After holding the position, repeat with the left arm.

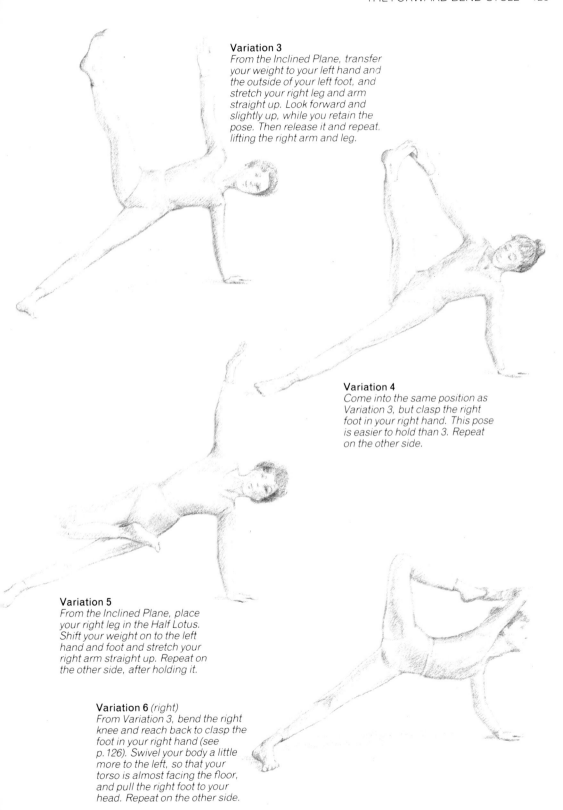

Variation 3
*From the Inclined Plane, transfer
your weight to your left hand and
the outside of your left foot, and
stretch your right leg and arm
straight up. Look forward and
slightly up, while you retain the
pose. Then release it and repeat,
lifting the right arm and leg.*

Variation 4
*Come into the same position as
Variation 3, but clasp the right
foot in your right hand. This pose
is easier to hold than 3. Repeat
on the other side.*

Variation 5
*From the Inclined Plane, place
your right leg in the Half Lotus.
Shift your weight on to the left
hand and foot and stretch your
right arm straight up. Repeat on
the other side, after holding it.*

Variation 6 *(right)*
*From Variation 3, bend the right
knee and reach back to clasp the
foot in your right hand (see
p. 126). Swivel your body a little
more to the left, so that your
torso is almost facing the floor,
and pull the right foot to your
head. Repeat on the other side.*

The Backward Bend Cycle

Having stretched the spine in the Forward Bend Cycle, you now compress the spinal vertebrae and stretch the entire front of your body, opening up the chest and abdomen and facilitating deep breathing. People sometimes become so absorbed by the backward bends that they start to practise them to the exclusion of other asanas. To keep your spine healthy, you must maintain a balance between forward and backward bends. In fact, after a particularly intense session of backward bends it is advisable to spend a little time in a forward bend, to bring the spine back to neutral. Another common mistake is to bend exclusively from one area of the spine – usually the lower back. Make sure that you always come into and out of the asanas slowly and with control, so that you can feel the movement spreading right from your neck to the base of your spine.

Cobra Variations

Once your back muscles have developed and your spine has become sufficiently flexible, you can comfortably hold Bhujang-asana with little support from your arms. Now you are ready to lift your arms up and use your hands to grip your knees or feet and pull your body even further back. These variations give the upper back a most satisfying stretch and, curling the body round, make a complete circuit for the flow of prana.

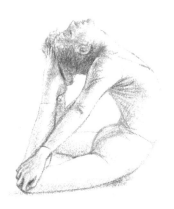

Variations 1 and 2
1 *From the full Cobra, move one hand to the centre in front of you. Reach back with the other hand and clasp your knee. Thus supported, stretch the first hand back to clasp the other knee. Pull on your knees and exhale to increase the curve of your spine. Reverse these steps to come out of the variations.*
2 *(right) Supporting yourself on one hand, reach back with the other and clasp both feet, using the handhold on page 126. Now reach back with the first hand and grip each foot in its respective hand. Pull your feet up.*

Locust Variations

In these variations, you project the body forward, lengthening spine and legs, rather than thrusting the legs upward, as in the Locust. You can try these poses as soon as you can hold Salabhasana without needing to support your weight with your arms. Here the arms push your legs out from the hips and bend the body backward from the upper spine and neck. Before you come into these variations pull your arms and shoulders away from your head, and push your chin forward along the floor; this will increase the stretch on your spine and reduces the pressure. Release the poses slowly, transferring your weight from your legs back to your arms.

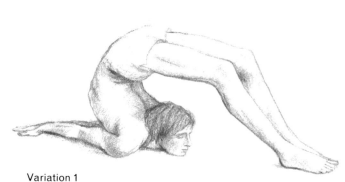

Variation 1
Bring your legs together and extend them beyond your head. When your feet eventually reach the floor, transfer some of your weight to them.

Variation 2 *(right)*
Separate your legs and stretch them out in front of you, pushing your heels forward. Bring your legs together once they are horizontal. To balance, you must pull your hips back just far enough to offset the weight of your legs.

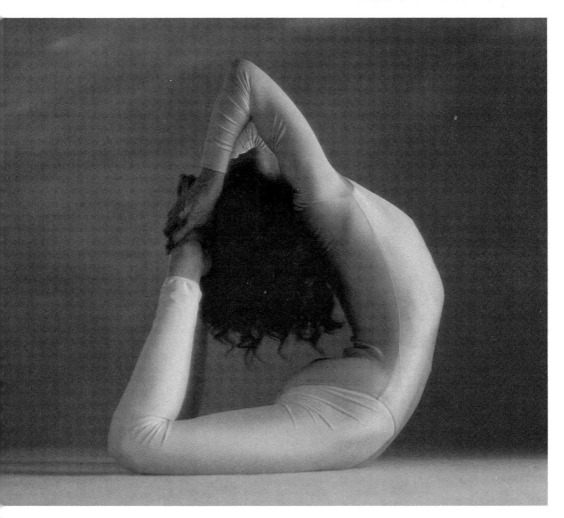

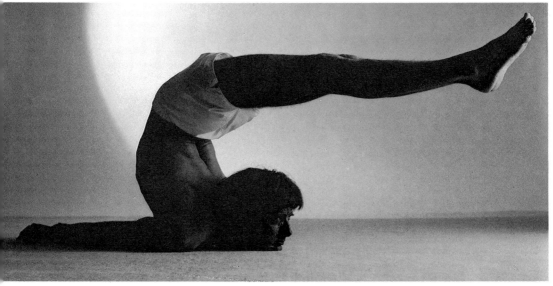

Backward Bend Handhold

This handhold is used for several asanas, including the Bow and Pigeon. Stretch the right hand out to the side, palm down. Turn the hand over to the right, so that the palm faces up and the thumb points behind you. Now, turning your body a little to the right, bring the arm back and clasp the outside of your right foot in your right hand, thumb on the sole, fingers on top. Bending your elbow turn it out and up and pull your foot forward. Repeat with left hand (and foot) if the pose calls for both.

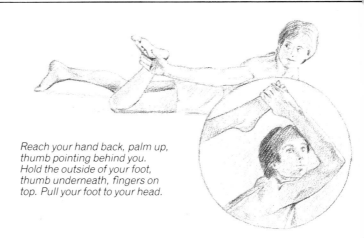

Reach your hand back, palm up, thumb pointing behind you. Hold the outside of your foot, thumb underneath, fingers on top. Pull your foot to your head.

Bow Variations

If you have ever wished you could pick your body up in both hands and reshape it at will, these variations come close to fulfilling that dream. Simply by pulling on your legs you have the power to change the nature of the backward bend and bring together parts of the body that normally never meet. In Variation 3, for example, you draw your feet down to your shoulders, while in 1 your heels come to rest on your forehead, leaving you to gaze up at the soles of your feet. The main difference between these variations and the basic Dhanurasana (p.54) lies in the handhold and arm position, shown above. This makes your arm-reach shorter and so gives the body a far more powerful stretch than the straight-armed grip. With your feet clasped securely in your hands, you can steer your legs forward or upward with great control – as if throwing a ball in slow motion. As you grow more supple, move your hands to your ankles or shins to draw the bowstrings tighter, and bring your knees together. This will intensify the stretch.

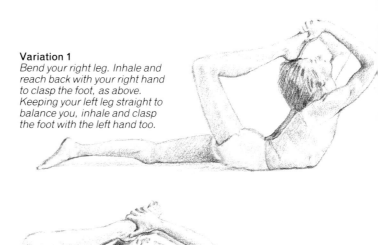

Variation 1
Bend your right leg. Inhale and reach back with your right hand to clasp the foot, as above. Keeping your left leg straight to balance you, inhale and clasp the foot with the left hand too.

Variation 2
Using the handhold above, come into the Bow. Breathing deeply, pull your feet a little further forward on each exhalation. In time you will be able to extend them beyond your head.

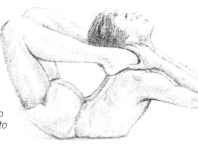

Variations 3 and 4
3 *(far right) After adopting Variation 1, try to straighten your arms and legs upward.*
4 *To master Poorna Dhanurasana, your shoulders must be relaxed. Hold Variation 1 for long enough to warm the body up. Then pull your feet gently down to your shoulders, keeping your head tilted back.*

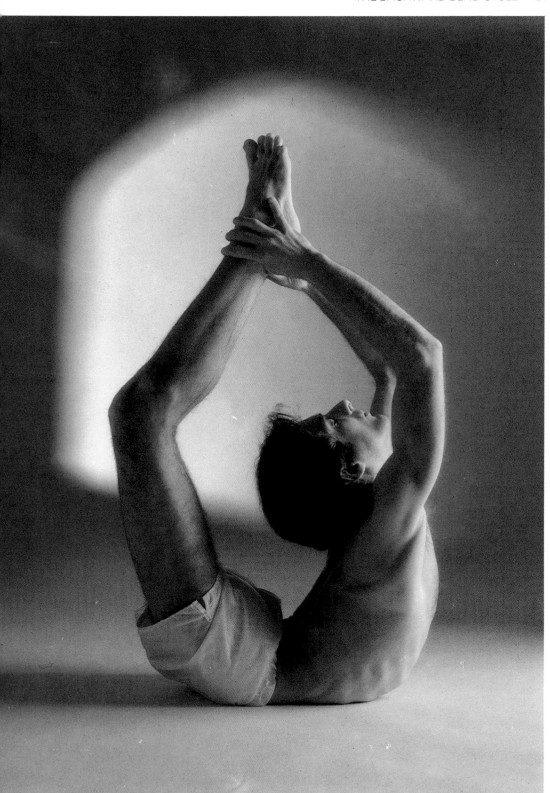

The Wheel

"He who practises this Asana will have perfect control of his body," Swami Sivananda said. The Wheel or Chakrasana is a most dynamic backward bend, stimulating all the chakras or energy centres and leaving you wonderfully exhilarated. To start with, you should practise pushing up into the pose from the floor, unless you are already very supple. When you first learn to arch backward into the pose from a standing position, you want to minimize the distance you have to drop down. Bring your body as low as possible by spreading your legs wide apart and bending your knees. Most important, centre your weight in your knees as you arch back – this way you will fall on your knees if you do by any chance lose your balance. Place your hands and feet the same distance apart to hold the pose steadily – think of your body as a table with four legs well placed. With time, you will bring your hands and feet together to complete the circle, as below right.

Alternative step into the Wheel

With feet far apart and hands on hips, arch slowly backward. Keep your weight in your knees and push your hips forward. Inhale, raise your arms over and behind your head and drop back onto your hands. To stand up again, shift your weight to your knees, then push yourself forward and bring your arms up one at a time or both at once.

Variation 1

Bending backward; gradually walk your hands down the back of your legs. When you reach your limit, thrust your hips forward and hold the pose. You can also use this variation to come into the basic Wheel: gripping one leg firmly, raise the other arm over your head and bring the hand down. When steady, repeat with the other arm.

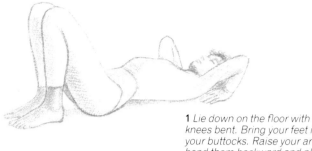

1 *Lie down on the floor with knees bent. Bring your feet in to your buttocks. Raise your arms, bend them backward and place your hands down behind your shoulders, fingers pointing toward your feet. Both feet and hands should be wide apart.*

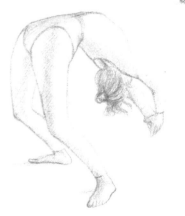

2 *Inhale, lift up your hips and, pressing down on your hands, place the top of your head on the floor. Rest briefly.*

3 *Inhale and straighten your arms, lifting your head as shown below. Raise your hips up high and breathe normally in the pose. With practice, you can walk your hands and feet closer together. If you are working on a blanket, clasp it in your hands and pull yourself back toward your feet. Reverse the steps to come down.*

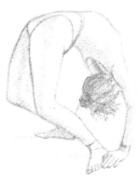

Variation 2 *(right)*

For Eka Pada Chakrasana, bring one leg to a central position to make a firm tripod. Inhale and lift the other leg, pushing up the heel. Let your raised leg elevate the entire body. Change legs.

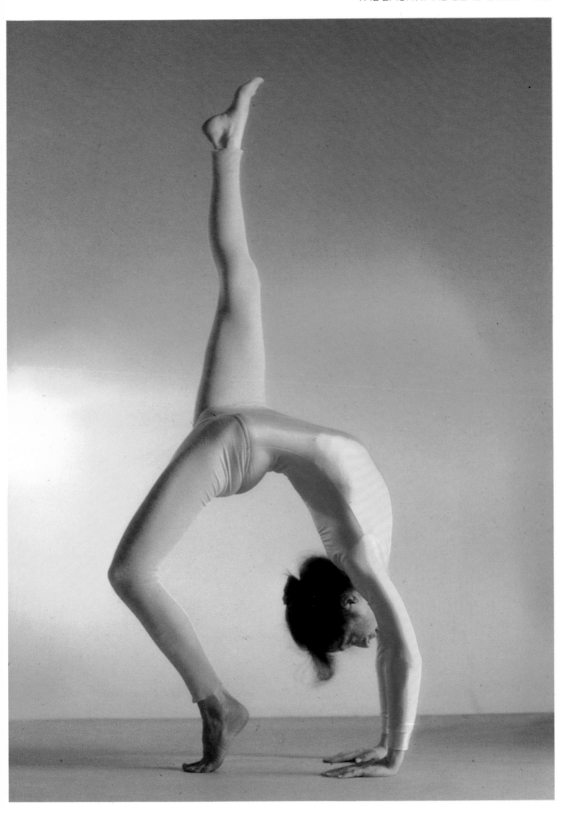

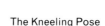

The Kneeling Pose

Supta Vajrasana prepares the body for the Diamond (below) by stretching the knees and thighs and encouraging a good lower back bend. When practising the position, make sure your shoulders and the back of your head rest on the floor and keep your knees as close together as possible, to obtain the fullest stretch. Allow your body to relax down toward the floor.

The Kneeling Pose
Kneel down and ease yourself back, using one elbow at a time, until you are lying on the floor. Fold your arms and place them above your head.

The Warrior

Many of us carry a lot of tension in our shoulders and upper backs. This not only causes bad posture and stiffness but also restricts the flow of prana. Veerasana opens up these areas, relaxing the muscles and allowing prana to flow freely. It also stretches the legs and makes the ankles flexible. If you are unable to clasp your hands at first, pull them nearer by holding a scarf between them.

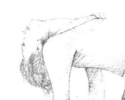

The Warrior
Kneel down with your right leg crossed over your left, heels in to the body, toes pointing outward. Keeping your back straight, reach up your back with your right arm and down over your shoulder with your left and clasp the hands together. Remain in the pose, pulling up with your left hand to increase the shoulder stretch. Repeat, reversing arms and legs.

The Kneeling Wheel

Both Chakrasana variation and the Diamond pose stretch the front of the body and build up strength in the abdominal muscles. To start with, practise it with your knees apart and release the pose one hand at a time. Keep your balance by leaning slightly away from the side of hand you are unclasping. As you advance, bring your legs closer together and let go of both ankles at once, allowing the forward push of your hips to carry you up.

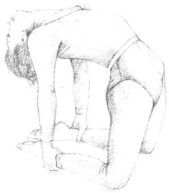

The Kneeling Wheel
Kneel down with your legs close together. Pushing forward with your hips, arch back and slightly to the right and clasp your right ankle. Now reach back to clasp the left ankle. Bend your head back in the position and breathe normally. Come out of the pose by pushing your weight forward, then inhaling and releasing your hands – either one at a time or both at once.

The Diamond

In this pose — Poorna Supta Vajrasana, and the variation opposite, you mould the body into a taut, self-contained diamond shape. If you cannot reach your feet in the pose pull on your blanket to ease your head nearer your feet. If you can clasp your feet, gently pull with your hands and push with your elbows to inch your head nearer your feet. Release these poses as slowly as possible, giving the body time to readjust.

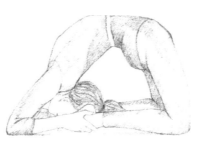

The Diamond and Variation
From the Kneeling Wheel, slowly arch back until your head rests on the floor. If your arch is high enough, clasp your feet or your ankles, using the handhold shown on page 126. Hold the pose, breathing deeply.

Variation *(right) From the above pose, stretch your hands forward to hold your knees. Try to increase the stretch with each exhalation by pulling the knees.*

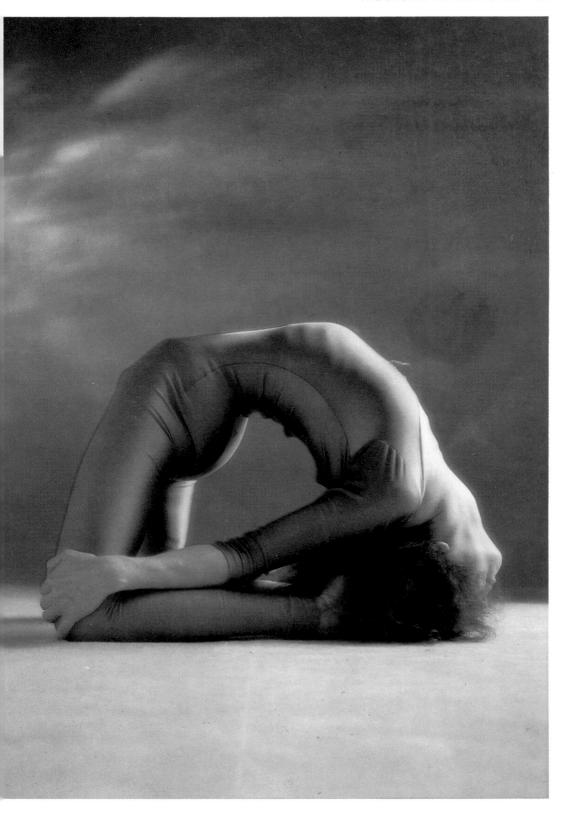

The Crescent Moon

In Anjaneyasana you curve the body into the shape of a crescent moon – often called the symbol of yoga. You need flexibility and a fairly good sense of balance to achieve the position, but unlike the Pigeon (below) you can have some experience of how the asana feels right from your early days of practice. Your weight is balanced on three points – the back knee and toes and the front foot. The back leg is the body's major support and gives you confidence to bend backward. To increase the stretch on your legs, keep the front foot flat, with the knee extended beyond it, and let your hips sink down toward the floor. This prepares you for the Splits (p. 140). Both the Crescent Moon and its variation expand the chest, so breathe deeply while holding the poses. Pull yourself back further on each exhalation. Be sure to perform these postures on both sides, reversing the leg positions.

The Pigeon

Here you thrust your chest right forward, like a pouter pigeon puffing out its breast. As a novice to the pose, you will find it easier to come into Kapotha Asana if you bend your body a little to the side of the raised back leg, then straighten up and face the front when you are balanced. Once you are more supple, you should dispense with this aid and reach back to hold your feet with both hands at once. The leg position shown right provides you with the most stable base. But you can also perform the pose with your front leg in an alternative position – in the Splits (p. 140); with the lower leg bent back on the outside instead of inside your thigh; or in the Crescent Moon, as featured on the opposite page. The longer you practise asanas, the more they seem to overlap. With eyes closed and a concentrated mind, you lose awareness of the distinctions between poses. All that you are conscious of is a feeling of lightness and energy.

The Crescent Moon *(above)*
Bend your left knee and stretch your right leg back, pushing the thigh down. Palms together, inhale and arch back, stretching your arms and head back.

Variation 1 *(right)*
Bring your legs into the Crescent Moon pose, top left. Then clasp your back foot, proceeding as for the Pigeon pose (bottom).

Variation 2 *(above)*
Bring your legs into the pose shown above left. Inhale, clasp your hands behind you and stretch them back over your leg until you reach your maximum bend. Now hold the leg and pull yourself back further.

1 *Sit down with your left foot in to your perineum and your right leg stretched straight out behind you. Bend your right leg and catch hold of the foot, as described on page 126.*

2 *Using your left hand to balance you, pull the foot up with your right hand and arch backward, bringing your head back toward the sole of your foot.*

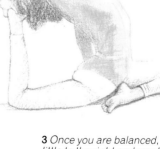

3 *Once you are balanced, lean a little to the right and reach back with the left hand also to clasp the foot. Now swivel your chest back to the front again. Repeat, reversing the legs.*

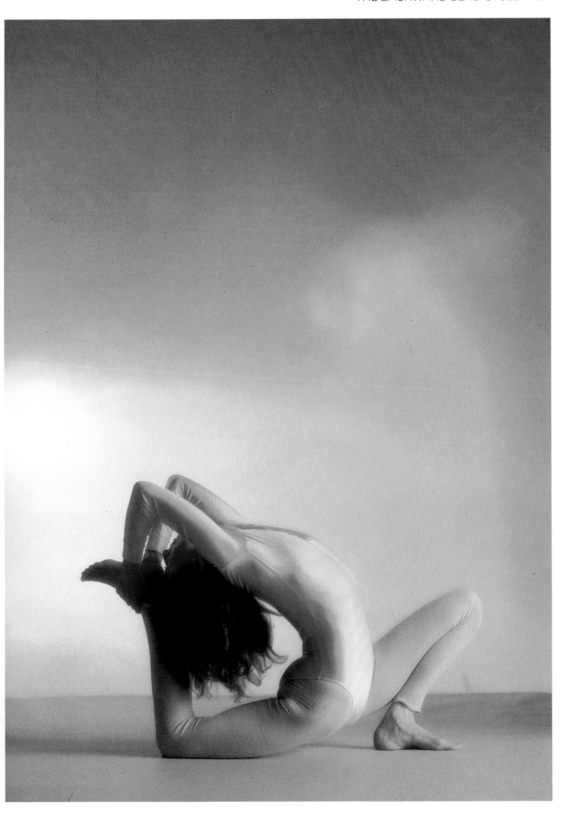

The Sitting Cycle

This cycle encompasses a wide variety of asanas – from Spinal Twists and Lotus variations to Shooting Bows and Splits. All of them focus particular attention on the legs, feet and hips and all originate from a basic seated position. This stable base frees you from the concerns of balancing or supporting the body, leaving you more energy to devote to the stretching, bending or twisting movements of the postures. However, due to such habits as sitting for long periods in chairs, and wearing shoes with raised heels, there is often some basic work to be done before you can fully enjoy these asanas. Even as an advanced student you will have to proceed gradually to remove the stiffness caused by years of unwise eating and improper exercise. But if you practise persistently and take care with your diet (pp. 78-85) you will succeed in easing the tightness and reap the full benefits of this cycle.

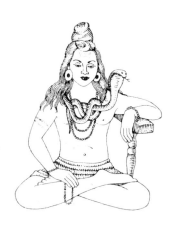

The Spinal Twist

Practising Matsyendrasana and its variations is very refreshing after the forward and backward bends, and encourages great flexibility in the spine. As in many of the sitting asanas, you use both the floor and parts of your body as levers – pulling on your ankles, pushing the backs of your arms against your knees to increase the stretch. As you twist your torso around, imagine you are wringing out a wet cloth. This squeezing movement stimulates circulation to the spine and prevents stagnation in the internal organs, ridding the body of toxins and breaking down fatty tissue. Prana suffuses the entire spinal area, giving you added strength and concentration. In the Half Spinal Twist (p. 56) you learnt the importance of keeping the spine erect. This becomes even more essential in these advanced asanas, as the twist is more extreme. Try to reach right up with your spine while rotating the body. Breathe normally as you hold these poses, twisting further into the position on every exhaled breath. Be sure to repeat each asana in the opposite direction, to obtain an equal twist on the other side.

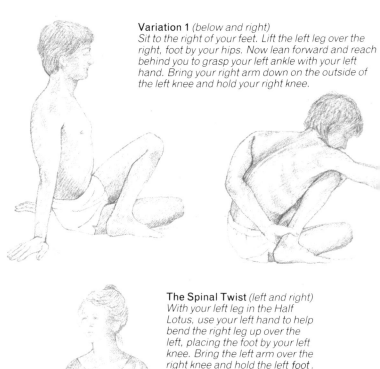

Variation 1 *(below and right)*
Sit to the right of your feet. Lift the left leg over the right, foot by your hips. Now lean forward and reach behind you to grasp your left ankle with your left hand. Bring your right arm down on the outside of the left knee and hold your right knee.

The Spinal Twist *(left and right)*
With your left leg in the Half Lotus, use your left hand to help bend the right leg up over the left, placing the foot by your left knee. Bring the left arm over the right knee and hold the left foot, twisting to the right.

Variation 2 *(far right)*
Come into the Spinal Twist. Then, as in Variation 1, reach back with the right hand and clasp the right ankle. A folded blanket under the buttock of the raised leg helps initially.

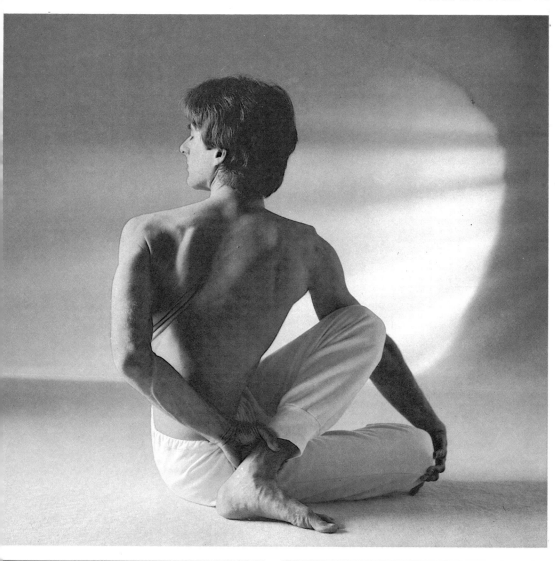

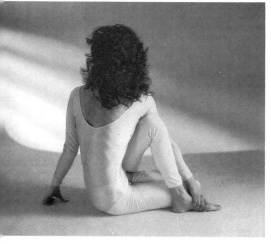

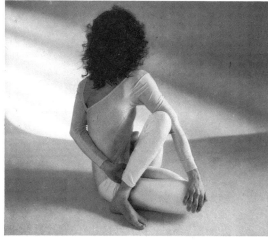

Lotus Variations

The Lotus, Padmasana, is a marvellously versatile pose that can be combined with a great variety of asanas. It elevates any asana of which it is a part, stilling the mind and thus increasing your power to control your body. In the Lotus your legs are folded into a small, easily manageable unit, giving you a solid foundation to sit on and a compact mass to lift up into the air. Once again, you are using both the floor and your own limbs as levers in these variations, to coax the body into positions of rare complexity, such as the Foetus and Bound Lotus. The Yoga Mudra tones the spinal nerves and is of great benefit to the proper functioning of the digestive system. Both this pose and the Bound Lotus help to awaken the dormant Kundalini. Although Variation 1 is not strictly a sitting pose, we have included it here to dissolve the boundaries that may exist in your mind between asanas from different cycles. Any asana or variation includes elements from more than one cycle – the "Lotus Scorpion" can be seen as a Headstand variation, a balancing pose and a sitting pose. The classic Lotus is performed with the left leg on top. But for the sake of balance you should repeat each of these variations with the right leg on top too. You will feel the difference at the base of your spine when you alter the leg position.

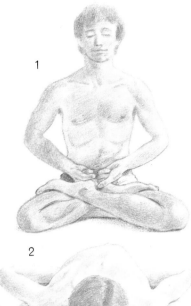

1

2

Lotus Variation 1 (right)
Come up into the Lotus Headstand. Now proceed as for the Scorpion. Don't worry about falling – your reflexes will automatically free the top leg first.

The Yoga Mudra (left)
1 Keeping the spine erect, make two fists and place them behind your heels, thumbs out. Press them gently but firmly into the lower abdomen. Inhale.
2 Exhaling, bend forward and bring your head down to the floor. Hold the pose. With deep abdominal breathing your fists, pressed by your heels, massage the internal organs.

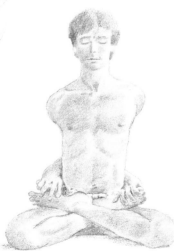

The Bound Lotus

Exhaling, twist slightly to the right and reach back with the right hand to grasp your right big toe. Inhale. Exhaling, twist slightly to the left and reach back with your left hand to grasp your left big toe. Straighten the body and breathe deeply. This is Bandha Padmasana.

Lotus Variation 2
With your legs in the Lotus, use your hands to raise yourself onto your knees, then to lie down on your front. Pause at this point, if necessary, with your head resting on your folded arms (p.106). Then place your hands palms down under your shoulders and proceed as for the Cobra (p.50). Keep your hips on the floor.

The Cock
For Kukutasana, sit in the Lotus. Now insert your hands between your calves and your thighs. Breathe in and press your palms down, pulling your legs up your arms. Keep your torso as straight as you can.

The Foetus
For Garbhasana, insert your hands between your legs, as above, bringing the elbows through to the other side and raising the legs. Bend your elbows, pulling your legs up toward your chest and clasp your ears, as shown far right.

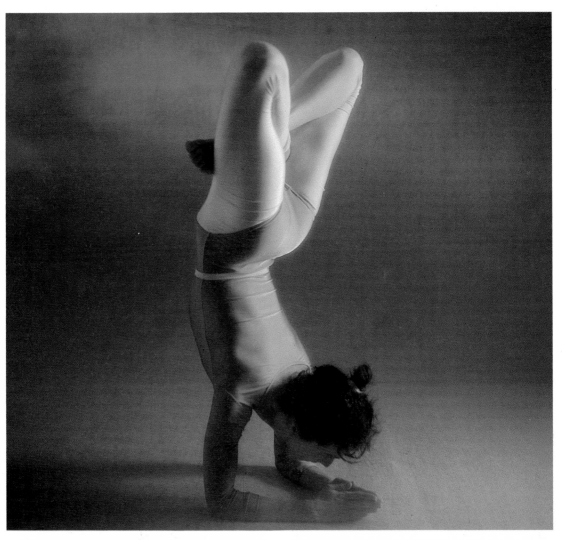

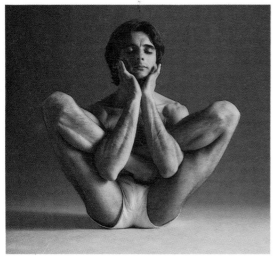

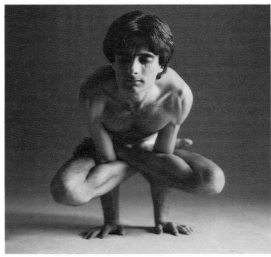

The Shooting Bow

In Akarna Dhanurasana, you draw one leg right back, like an archer drawing a bow. In fact, from the classic position (top) you can exhale and release the leg like an arrow, shooting it forward, heel first. In all these asanas, one side of the body maintains a forward bend while you open up the hip and shoulder joints on the other side. The leg muscles are stretched and both arms and legs strengthened, making the Shooting Bow a useful preliminary to the Leg behind Head Pose (below). Try to straighten the body up and look to the front while you hold these poses, and breathe slowly and deeply — this not only helps you to pull your leg further back, but also enables you to balance much more easily.

Variation 1
Come into the pose, but pull the right foot up above your head and straighten the leg.

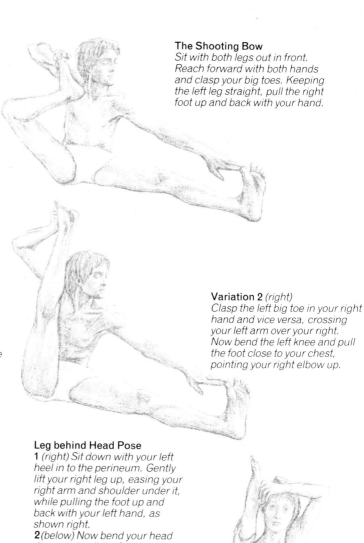

The Shooting Bow
Sit with both legs out in front. Reach forward with both hands and clasp your big toes. Keeping the left leg straight, pull the right foot up and back with your hand.

Variation 2 *(right)*
Clasp the left big toe in your right hand and vice versa, crossing your left arm over your right. Now bend the left knee and pull the foot close to your chest, pointing your right elbow up.

Leg behind Head Pose

To prepare your body for these asanas, try this warm-up first. Bend the right leg and bring it up parallel to your chest. Cradle the lower leg in your arms and rock it from side to side. Now, clasping the ankle, bring the sole of the foot to your chest, then raise the foot and touch the toes to your forehead, then to your ear. Repeat with the left leg. With practice, you will bring the leg behind your head and can work toward bringing more of your body in front of your leg. Eventually the leg will come right back behind your shoulder. Then you will no longer need to hold your leg in place with your hands. You can also approach the pose from a lying down position, which makes it easier. This asana exerts great pressure on the abdominal organs. Lift the right leg first, to massage the ascending colon, then the left leg, to massage the descending colon. The order is important.

Leg behind Head Pose
1 *(right)* Sit down with your left heel in to the perineum. Gently lift your right leg up, easing your right arm and shoulder under it, while pulling the foot up and back with your left hand, as shown right.
2 *(below)* Now bend your head down and pull the foot back behind your head and shoulder. Bring your palms together in the prayer pose. This is Eka Pada Sirasana.

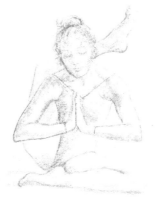

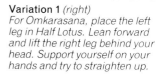

Variation 1 *(right)*
For Omkarasana, place the left leg in Half Lotus. Lean forward and lift the right leg behind your head. Support yourself on your hands and try to straighten up.

Variation 2 *(far right)*
For Dwipada Sirasana, lie on your back and bring first one leg then the other behind your head, crossing your ankles.

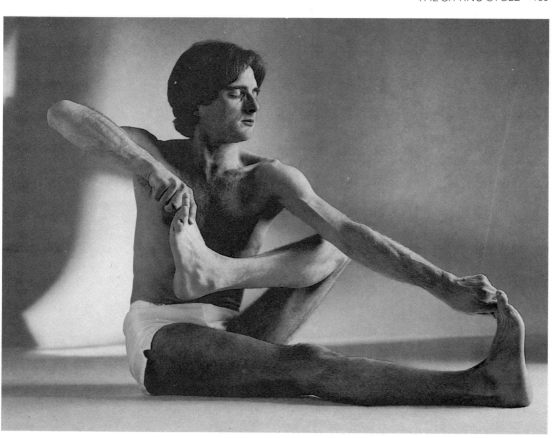

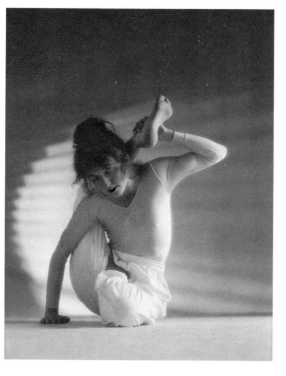

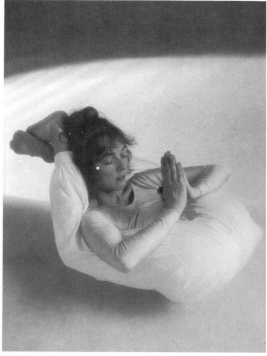

The Splits

The only way to master Anjaney-asana, the Splits is by constant repetition. If you try it once a year you will never succeed, but if you incorporate it in your daily set of asanas, your legs will gradually ease apart. If it seems an extreme pose, it may inspire you to know that the legs are capable of an even greater stretch – with both back and front legs lifted some way off the floor, knees straight. Once you are comfortable in the Splits, the pose brings you a wonderful feeling of balance and symmetry. It is a very stable asana, providing the longest base that your body can rest on. The Splits opens the door to many other poses – some of the advanced inverted or balancing poses become more accessible when you can reach your leg down or raise it up into them. And because practising the Splits improves the circulation in your legs, it is of great benefit to all standing poses. As soon as you have mastered both the Pigeon and the Splits, you can combine the two and practise Variation 3. This asana will show up any asymmetry between your two sides and give you a chance to rectify it – for example, if your right side is more flexible, pull a little bit more when holding the left foot. Once you can do this variation, you need no longer practise the Pigeon with any other leg position, since pressing the front leg straight down in the Splits gives you the most complete backward bend.

1 *Supporting your weight on your hands, stretch one leg forward to rest on the heel and the other back, keeping the knee up.*

2 *Gradually take less of your weight on your hands, bouncing gently up and down to stretch the legs further apart. Once you can rest both legs flat on the floor, bring your palms together in the prayer pose.*

Variation 4
Clasp the toes of your left foot with your left hand. Now bend the right knee and reach back to clasp the foot in your right hand.

Variation 1 (below)
In the Splits, with your hands in the prayer pose, inhale. Now exhale and, leading with the hands, bend forward from the waist and come down over the front leg.

Variation 2 (right)
With your legs in the Splits and your hands in the prayer pose, inhale. Now exhale and arch back, bringing your arms over your head. Use your breathing to keep your balance in the position and to focus your mind.

Variation 3
Bend your right knee; reach back and clasp the foot with the right hand (as on p. 126). Now pull the foot to your head and hold it with your left hand too.

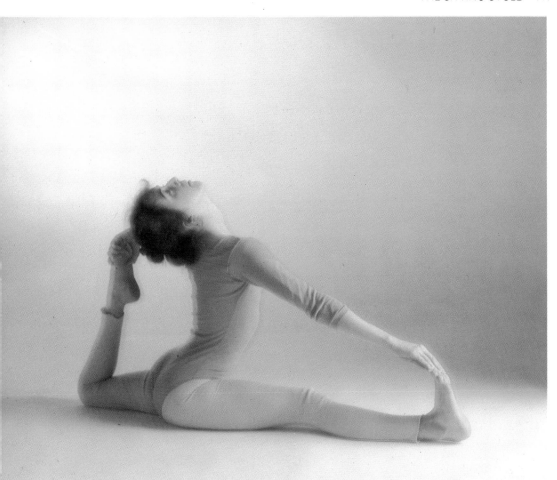

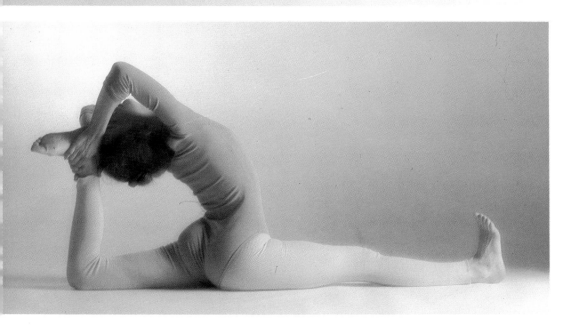

The Balancing Cycle

It is easiest to balance if you can distribute your weight over a wide area or a number of points, as in the Headstand "tripod". When you need to balance on one leg or on your hands, the secret lies in multiplying your points of support. In the Tree, for example, think of yourself as having two points of balance rather than one – let your weight alternate between your heels and toes initially, until you find your equilibrium. As for all asanas, bare feet are essential since you need to be able to spread your toes out and grip the floor in order to hold steady. While practising the balancing poses, fix your gaze on one spot – a mark on the wall, perhaps, or a speck of dust on the floor. Like a sailor throwing a line to shore, mentally cast a thread to that spot so that you can hold on to it with your mind.

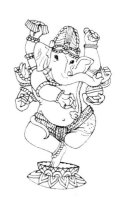

The Peacock

Balancing in Mayoorasana, the Peacock, demands strength and total concentration. When the asana is performed correctly, head, body and legs make a straight line, parallel with the floor. The pose is highly bene-ficial for the digestion – even before you can balance on your hands – as the weight of the body presses the elbows into the upper abdomen, massaging the pancreas and spleen. Once you are proficient at this asana, you can try practising it with a more advanced hand position. Either use two fists, or place your hands down with your fingertips pointing toward your head in-stead of backward.

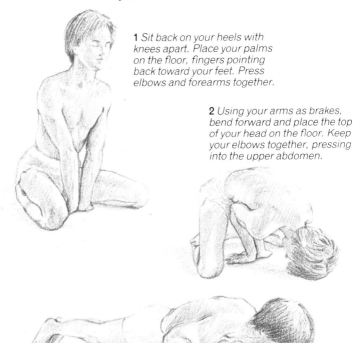

1 *Sit back on your heels with knees apart. Place your palms on the floor, fingers pointing back toward your feet. Press elbows and forearms together.*

2 *Using your arms as brakes, bend forward and place the top of your head on the floor. Keep your elbows together, pressing into the upper abdomen.*

3 *(right) Stretch your legs back one at a time, keeping the knees off the floor and the feet together. Your weight should be on your toes, hands and head. Now lift your head.*

4 *(left) Inhale and gently ride forward on your arms, lifting your toes up and balancing on your hands. Keep your legs straight. Hold the pose as long as possible, breathing normally; then exhale and release it, coming down on your toes.*

Variation 1 *(right)*
Come into the Peacock pose, as described above. But in step 3, instead of lifting your head, rest your chin on the floor, then raise both legs up vertically, as in the Locust. It is in this position that the pose resembles a peacock displaying his tail feathers.

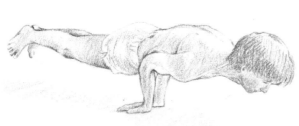

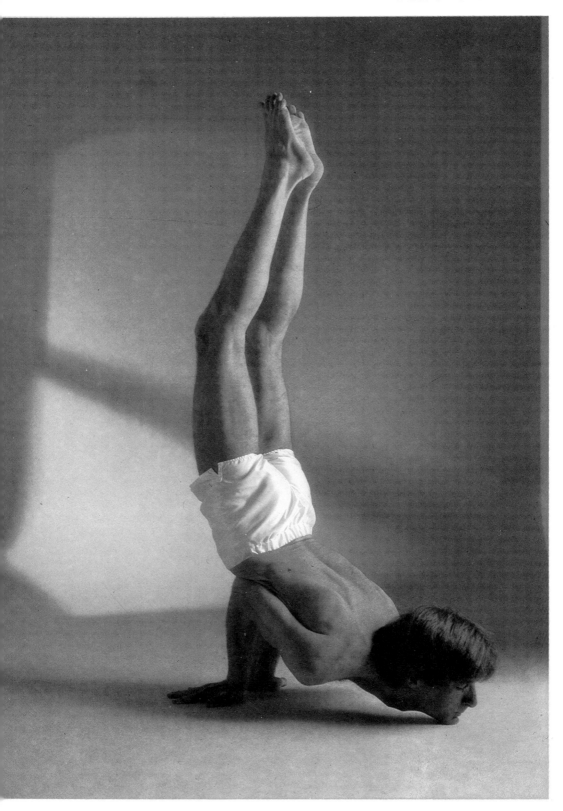

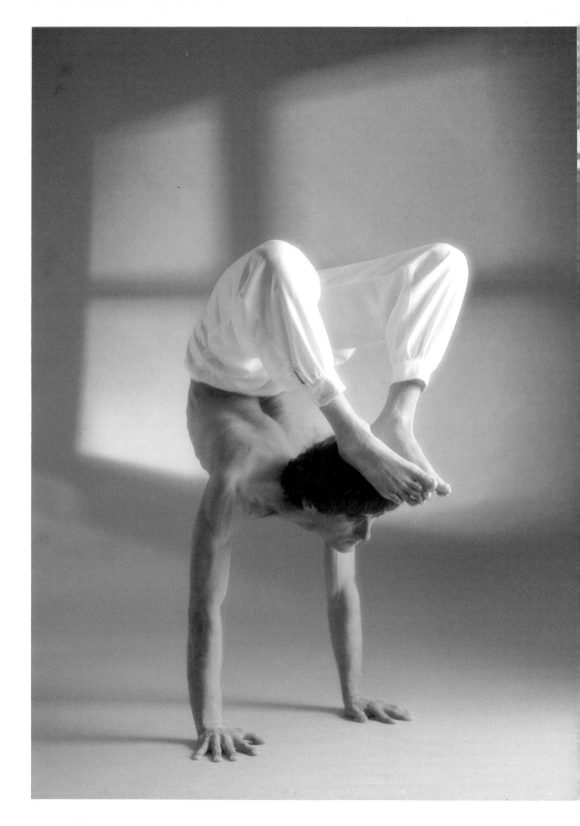

The Handstand

Like the Scorpion, taming the Handstand – Vrikshasana – is as much a matter of positive thinking as of balance. Think of your arms as legs, and spread your fingers out to give yourself a broader foundation and grip the floor. Try practising the asana against a wall initially, if you are scared of falling. Come up into the pose with your elbows straight and your hands at least two feet from the wall, letting your feet drop over on to it. Then lift your feet off and balance for a few moments, so that you begin to experience how it feels to be free-standing. As soon as you have gained confidence, dispense with the wall. In time you will even be able to walk a few steps on your hands.

Crow Variations

These positions are far simpler to perform than they look. The secret is to make a steady shelf with your arms to support the weight of your legs. Once you have mastered the basic Kakasana (p.60) you can develop the strength of your torso by working on one side of the body at a time and trying to straighten your legs. You will find it easier to balance in Variations 1 and 3 if you remember to lean a little way to the opposite side from the one your legs are on. Always repeat these variations both to the left and right of your hands. Performing these poses helps to build up the strength in your arms and wrists necessary for the Handstand, as well as boosting your confidence in your ability to balance. With practice, you can even unfold your legs from the basic Crow and bring them up into the Handstand.

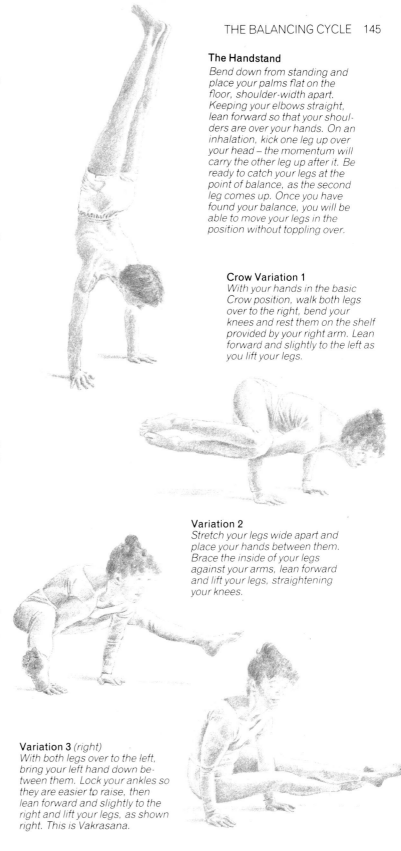

The Handstand
Bend down from standing and place your palms flat on the floor, shoulder-width apart. Keeping your elbows straight, lean forward so that your shoulders are over your hands. On an inhalation, kick one leg up over your head – the momentum will carry the other leg up after it. Be ready to catch your legs at the point of balance, as the second leg comes up. Once you have found your balance, you will be able to move your legs in the position without toppling over.

Crow Variation 1
With your hands in the basic Crow position, walk both legs over to the right, bend your knees and rest them on the shelf provided by your right arm. Lean forward and slightly to the left as you lift your legs.

Variation 2
Stretch your legs wide apart and place your hands between them. Brace the inside of your legs against your arms, lean forward and lift your legs, straightening your knees.

Handstand Variation *(left)*
Come up into the Handstand; then bend your knees, gradually bringing the feet down to your head. Keep your balance between the heels and fingers of your hands.

Variation 3 *(right)*
With both legs over to the left, bring your left hand down between them. Lock your ankles so they are easier to raise, then lean forward and slightly to the right and lift your legs, as shown right. This is Vakrasana.

The Eagle

This pose is named after Garuda, the mythical eagle (shown on p. 110) who had the beak and wings of a bird but the body of a man. Garuda Asana does for the arms and legs what the Spinal Twist does for the spine, twisting and squeezing first one side and then the other, to increase circulation to the limbs. It is an excellent remedy for varicose veins. Because the leg that supports your weight is bent this strengthens your leg muscles. Squeezing your arms and legs together while maintaining the position improves circulation and develops an awareness of your extremities, right up to your fingers and toes. Hold the pose, breathing deeply; then repeat, changing arms and legs.

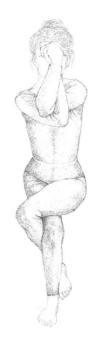

The Eagle
Stand on the right leg, knee slightly bent. Wrap the left leg around it so that the toes of the left foot are on the inside of the right ankle. Bring the right forearm in front of your face and wrap the left arm around it from inside, clasping the hands. Bend as low as you can and hold the position, squeezing arms and legs together.

The Tree

Practising this asana brings a wonderful feeling of inner peace. Poised on one leg with the other leg tucked securely in the Half Lotus and hands pressed together in the prayer pose, you can balance undisturbed by the body. In ancient times, yogis would remain in the Tree for days at a time as a form of "tapas" or austerity. Even today, many are to be found meditating in this pose on the banks of the Ganges and in other holy places. Practise the Tree in stages. Before placing your leg in the Half Lotus, first get your balance with the leg just raised, then with the foot pressed against the inner thigh of the opposite leg. (Pulling back with the standing leg will also help you to balance.) Breathe deeply while you hold the poses and repeat them on both sides. Standing up from a kneeling or a squatting Tree demands great concentration and control – release the asanas very slowly, using your breath to carry you up. As in all the balancing poses, fix your gaze on a point in front of you, to focus your concentration. Once you can hold the poses effortlessly, practise with eyes closed.

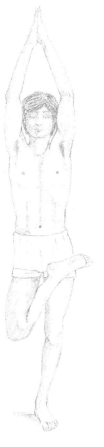

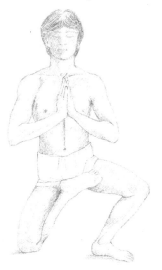

The Tree and Variations
For the classic pose left, place one leg in the Half Lotus. Join palms in the prayer pose, then raise them above your head.
One Knee and Foot Pose
(below) In Vatyanasana, bend the standing leg, lean slightly forward; come down on the other knee.
The Tiptoe Pose *In Padand-gushtasana (opposite) Bend the standing leg and gently sit down on your heel.*

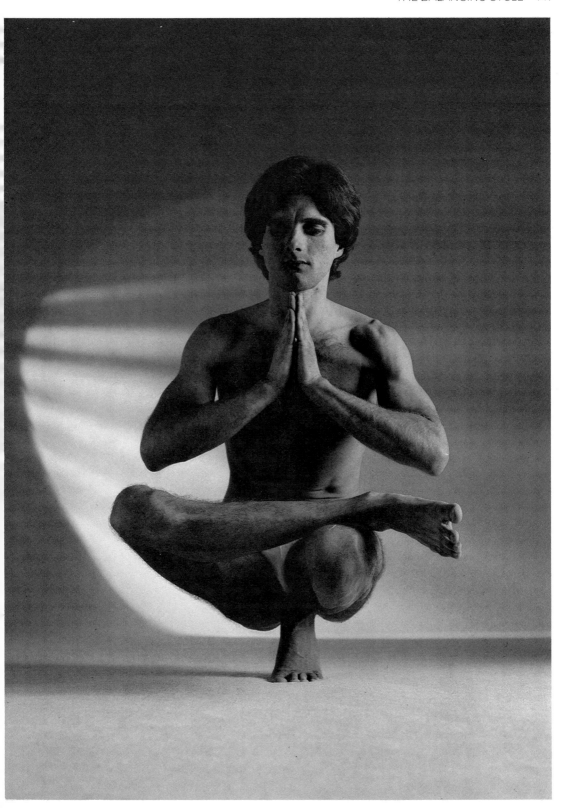

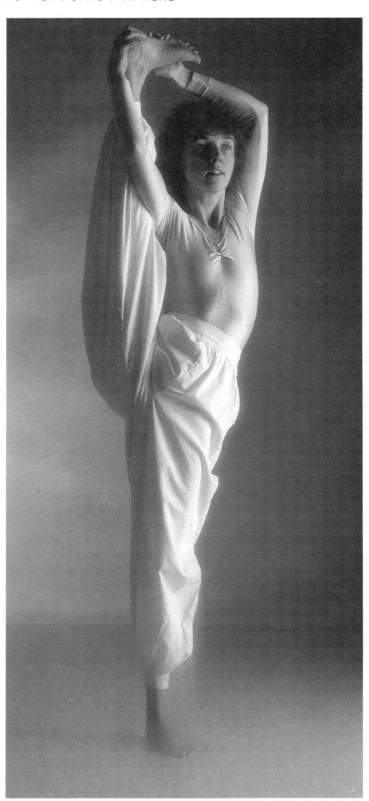

The Standing Splits

These Anjaneyasana variations are by nature both balancing poses and forward bends, sharing the benefits of both cycles. Unlike the sitting Splits, where gravity helps to increase the stretch, here you are working against gravity, using your arms to pull the raised leg up and carry its weight. Practising these asanas increases your strength, suppleness and sense of balance. Stretch the toes of your supporting foot out to grip the floor and give you a wider base. And, when coming into the poses, pull your legs up slowly and keep your mind concentrated. Push up with the standing leg and try to keep your legs and torso straight, lengthening your body up toward the ceiling.

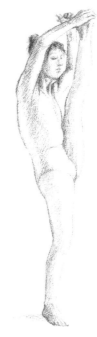

Standing Splits Variations
1 *Hold the left foot up with both hands, knee bent. Now straighten the knee and pull the leg in.*
2 *(left) Bend the left knee out to the side. Stretch your left hand along the inside leg and hold the heel. Straighten the leg and pull it up. Reach over your head with the right hand and pull the foot closer in to your head.*

Lord Nataraja Pose

Nataraja is one of the names given to Siva, the Cosmic Dancer, who is often depicted in this position. It is said that when Siva brings down his foot, the universe will be destroyed and a new world created. When you come into Natarajasana, or the variation, lean forward to help you pull the leg up, then try to straighten the body again. Keep the standing leg firm and straight to stabilize you. When your head is vertical, the emphasis is on an upward movement, while dropping the head back turns the pose into more of a backward bend and requires greater balance and control. In the classic pose just one hand holds the raised foot; but two hands achieve a fuller stretch.

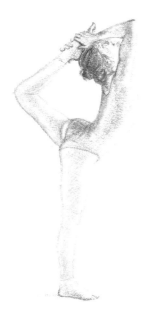

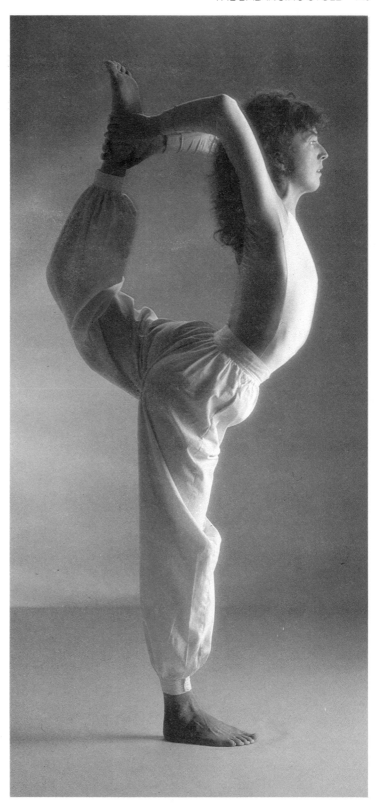

Natarajasana and Variation
Bend the left leg up behind you. Hold the ankle with the left hand (as on p.54) and pull up high. Change handhold (p.126) and reach back with the right hand also, to clasp the foot. Drop your head back on to the foot.
Variation *(right) Proceed as above, but rather than bringing head to foot, pull the foot above the head. Keep erect.*

The Standing Pose

These asanas demand – and develop – flexibility as well as strength. For this reason, you will find them easier to hold if you can already do the Splits. In the Standing Pose (top) you should try to create a straight line from your fingertips to your back foot, forming the body into a 'T' shape. In Variation 2, stretch your hands out away from each other and be sure to keep your back foot flat on the floor. You can use this pose to get into Variation 1. Lean over, bringing your chest to your thigh. Stretch both arms forward, then straighten the front leg and raise the back leg. Holding these poses will firm your legs, arms and hips when practised regularly. Don't forget to perform them on both sides.

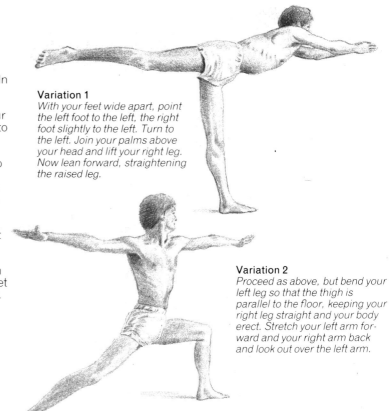

Variation 1
With your feet wide apart, point the left foot to the left, the right foot slightly to the left. Turn to the left. Join your palms above your head and lift your right leg. Now lean forward, straightening the raised leg.

Variation 2
Proceed as above, but bend your left leg so that the thigh is parallel to the floor, keeping your right leg straight and your body erect. Stretch your left arm forward and your right arm back and look out over the left arm.

Head to Feet Pose

As you develop your sense of balance, you will become more and more sensitive to the vital role played by the feet. If your feet are stiff and immobile, you will not be able to grip the floor well with your toes, nor stand correctly. Bringing your head to meet your feet in Pada Hasth-asana increases your aware-ness of these undervalued parts. Stretching your arms back helps you to balance and enables you to bend forward with your back straight.

Head to Feet Pose
Legs apart and hands clasped behind you, turn left. Now bend low, bringing chin down leg.

Variation
Spread your legs a little further apart, then proceed as above. But as you bend your body for-ward, bend the knee and try to bring your nose down to touch your toes. Straighten your arms.

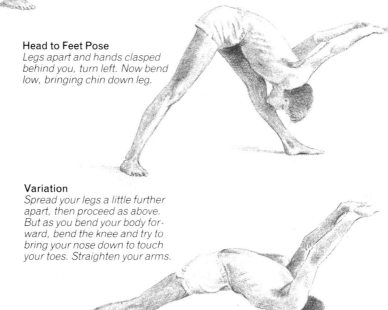

Triangle Variations

In order to achieve the freedom of movement needed for the more advanced asanas, it is important to keep the sides of the body stretched and toned. These Trikonasana variations lengthen and twist the sides and give the spine a powerful lateral stretch. Each of the poses is made up of three points – the extended hand, adjacent hand and foot, and the back foot. If you ran a thread between the points, you could create a triangle – hence their name. Here, once again, you are training your sense of balance – especially in Variations 1 and 3, when your legs face in the opposite direction to your torso. Make sure that your front thigh is parallel to the floor and your back leg straight in Variations 2 and 3. Repeat all the variations, giving equal time to both sides of the body.

Variation 1
Spread your legs about 3 feet apart, left foot pointing to the left, right foot pointing slightly to the left. Inhale. Exhaling, twist to the left and bend down, bringing your right palm down on the outside of the left foot. Stretch the left arm up and look at the fingertips of the left hand.

Variation 2
Bring your legs into position, as above, but a foot further apart. Now bend your left knee, bringing the left armpit down over it and place the left palm on the floor on the inside of your left foot. Stretch your right arm out alongside your right ear, making a straight line from the right hand to the right foot. Look up while holding the pose.

Variation 3
From Variation 2, swivel your body around to face the opposite direction, bringing the right armpit over the left knee and the right palm to the floor on the outside of your left foot. Stretch your left arm out by your left ear and look up.

The Cycles of Asanas

This chart provides an overview of all the asanas in the book which you should refer to when planning what to practise in your own set of asanas – just as you look at a map when deciding on your route through a country. The asanas from the Basic Session are illustrated in black, to show you how to incorporate the new poses into the basic pattern. The figures in pink represent the entirely new asanas taught in this Asanas and Variations section. All the variations of both basic and new asanas are described in shorthand fashion, each within its appropriate cycle. Naturally you will have to learn the new asanas and variations from the instructions given on the relevant page before you can use the shorthand versions here – these are intended purely as reminders of the poses, not as directions. No two bodies are the same – an asana that is simple for one student may demand more work for another. For this reason it is not possible to give an intermediate or advanced sequence. You should just proceed at your own pace, taking care always to balance the asanas you choose to practise.

The Headstand Cycle

(102-103)
Leg Raising Vars:
1 Double Leg Raising
2 Foot to palm swing
Headstand Leg Vars:
1 Legs to sides (Side Splits)
2 Leg lowered to front
3 As 1, leg lowered to side
4 Legs front and back

(104-105)
The Scorpion
Scorpion Vars:
1 Legs straight up
2 Legs horizontal
(106-107)
Headstand Arm Vars:
1 Elbows up, palms down
2 Arm(s) outstretched
3 Arms folded to head
(108-109)
Lotus Headstand:
Lotus in the Headstand
Var: *Legs in Lotus twist*
Single Leg Inverted Pose
1 Headstand Wheel with raised leg

The Shoulderstand Cycle

(110-111)
Shoulderstand Leg and Arm Vars:
1 Leg to floor
2 Leg bent, arm out
3 Arms up by hips (full Shoulderstand)
4 Eagle Shoulderstand: Legs twisted
5 Leg down, leg in Half Lotus (Half Lotus Plough)

(112-113)
Plough Vars:
1 Knees to the side
2 Knees behind head
3 Lotus Plough
Ear to Knee Pose

(114-115)
Bridge Vars:
1 Bridge with leg raised
2 Bridge with hips up, ankles held
3 Bridge in Lotus

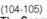
Fish Vars:
1 Lotus Fish
2 Bound Lotus Fish

The Forward Bend Cycle

(116-117)
The Forward Bend Vars:
1 Palms around soles, fingers under heels
2 Elbows on floor, fingers around arches
3 Arm clasping wrist beyond foot
4 Hands in prayer pose behind back
5 Balancing on buttocks
6 Forward Bend twist

(118-119)
Head to Knee Pose
Head to Knee Vars:
1 Hand behind back holding foot
2 Bending to the side, top arm back
3 Bending to the side, head on the floor
(120-121)
The Side Splits Twist Vars:
1 Hand behind back holding thigh; torso along leg
2 Both hands to feet, back along leg
Leg and Arm Stretching Vars:
1 Legs out, body forward (Forward Bend in Side Splits)
2 Legs out, body forward, hands to feet

The Tortoise
The Balancing Tortoise:
Ankles behind head, balancing on hands

(122-123)
The Inclined Plane
Inclined Plane Vars:
1 Leg raising
2 Arm raising
3 Leg and arm raising
4 Leg and arm raising, hand holding foot
5 Leg and arm raising in Half Lotus
6 Hand holding raised leg over head (Inclined Plane with Natarajasana)

The Backward Bend Cycle

(124-125)
Cobra Vars:
*1 Hands to knees
2 Hands holding feet*

Locust Vars:
*1 Feet to floor
2 Legs horizontal*

(126-127)
Bow Vars:
*1 One leg held, one
straight out (Half Bow)
2 Feet beyond head
3 Feet behind head, arms
and legs upward
4 Feet to shoulders*

(128-129)
The Wheel
Wheel Vars:
*1 Hands on back of legs
2 One leg raised (Eka
Pada Chakrasana)*

(130-131)
The Kneeling Pose

The Warrior
The Kneeling Wheel:
*On knees, clasping
ankles*

The Diamond
Diamond Var:
Hands holding knees

(132-133)
Crescent Moon

Crescent Moon Vars:
*1 Clasping back feet
(as in Pigeon)
2 Arms stretched
back over leg*

The Pigeon

The Sitting Cycle

(134-135)
The Spinal Twist
Spinal Twist Vars:
*1 Holding ankle
2 Holding ankle behind
back in Half Lotus*

(136-137)
Lotus Vars:
*1 Lotus with Scorpion
2 Lotus in Cobra position*
The Yoga Mudra:
*Fists into abdomen,
bending forward*
The Bound Lotus:
*Hands holding toes
behind back*

The Cock

The Foetus

(138-139)
The Shooting Bow

*1 Foot straight above
head
2 Hands holding
opposite feet*

The Leg Behind Head Pose
Leg Behind Head Vars:
*1 Lower leg in Half Lotus
2 Lying on back, both
legs behind head*

*1 Forward bending
2 Hands in prayer pose,
backward bending
3 Back foot to head, arm
to front toe
4 As 3, holding bent
back leg (Pigeon Splits)*

The Balancing Cycle

(142-143)
The Peacock
Peacock Var:
*Legs raised in Locust,
chin on floor*
(144-145)

The Handstand
Handstand Var:
*Feet to head
(Handstand Scorpion)*
Crow Vars:
*1 Side Crow, legs to side
2 Legs wide apart
3 Side Crow, arm be-
tween legs*

(146-147)
The Eagle

The Tree
One Knee and Foot Pose:
Knee to floor in Half Lotus
The Tiptoe Pose:
*Half Lotus, resting on
heel*
(149-149)
Standing Splits Vars:
*1 Leg up in front, hand
holding foot
2 Leg up at side, arm
over head holding foot*

Lord Nataraja
Natarajasana Var:
*Head, neck and spine
straight*

(150-151)
Standing Pose

Standing Pose Vars:
*1 Stretch balancing on
one leg
2 Arm and leg stretching*

The Head to Feet Pose
Head to Feet Var:
*Legs apart, knee bent,
head to toe*

Triangle Vars:
*1 Twisting backward
2 Legs further apart,*

*knee under arm
3 As 2, twisting backward*

Kriyas

The Yogi regards his body as a vehicle in which he is evolving toward higher consciousness. To run smoothly, this vehicle must be cleansed both internally and externally – just as we wash our hands, we should also keep the internal passage-ways clean – after all, they are continuations of the outer covering of skin. The six kriyas are purification practices which cleanse or tone the parts of the body we often neglect. They consist of: Kapalabhati (p.72); Tratak (pp.95-97); Neti, which clears the nasal passages; Dhauti, which is mainly for the digestive tract and includes Kunjar Kriya (p.86) and Agni Sara (p.182), and Vastra Dhauti, shown below; Nauli, which tones the abdominal viscera; and Basti, which washes out the colon. By removing toxins from the system, the kriyas – when practised regularly – make the mind sharp and the senses keen, and increase the body's resistance to disease.

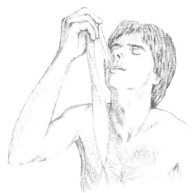

Neti
Neti should be performed daily, standing in front of a mirror, with the head tilted back so that you can see the opening's, just inside the nostrils. There are two methods. In Sutra Neti, you pass a catheter or a 12-inch piece of waxed cord into one nostril and out through the mouth, then repeat on the other side. It may take a little practice to make sure the cord comes out of your mouth, rather than going up your nostril or down your throat. In Jala Neti, you use a small pot with a spout to pour lightly salted water in one nostril and out of the other. If the other nostril is blocked, the water will flow down into your mouth and you can spit it out. After performing it on both sides, blow any excess water out, one side at a time.

Sutra Neti
Dip the cord in lukewarm salty water. Insert it into the hole just inside your nostril. When you see the tip emerging at the back of your mouth, reach in and slowly pull it out.

Jala Neti
With your head tilted to the left, pour water into your right nostril and out of the left (or out of your mouth).

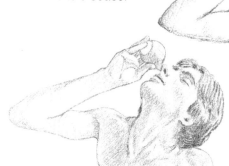

Vastra Dhauti
Dip the gauze in lukewarm salty water. While sipping water, slowly swallow the gauze. Go as far as you can, then gently ease it back up and out of your mouth.

Vastra Dhauti
Yogis practise this once a week, first thing in the morning on an empty stomach. It involves swallowing a 15-foot strip of hemmed gauze, then gently pulling it out, to remove accumulated mucous and waste from the stomach and oesophagus. At first you may feel nauseous and only succeed in swallowing an inch or two. But if you practise taking in a few more inches each day, in time you will be able to swallow the full length. After practising it you should drink a glass of milk. Vastra Dhauti requires the supervision of a qualified yoga teacher.

Nauli

Here you rotate the central abdominal muscle in a churning motion. This takes concentration as well as control, as you are learning to manipulate an involuntary muscle. It helps therefore if you focus on your abdomen while doing Nauli. Practising Agni Sara (p. 182) will prepare you for the exercise. Start by trying to isolate the muscle so that it forms a vertical ridge down the centre of your abdomen. Then practise pushing down with your left hand and moving the muscle to the right, and vice versa. Eventually, you will achieve a smooth, wave-like motion, most invigorating for the internal organs. This tones the stomach, intestines and liver, relieves menstrual problems, and increases the flow of prana.

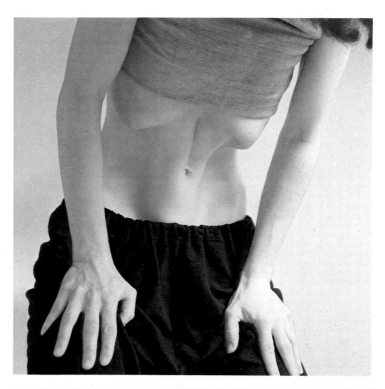

Nauli *(right)*
Stand with your legs apart, knees slightly bent, hands on thighs. Exhale and perform Uddiyana Bandha. Contract the sides of the abdomen, isolating the central muscle (above). Now press on alternate hands to move the muscle from one side to the other (below)

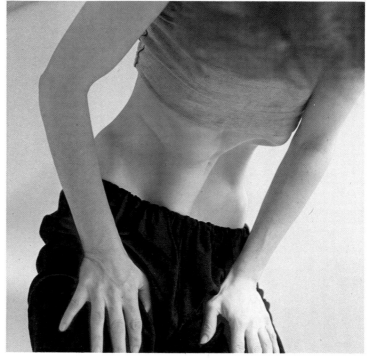

Basti

This is a natural method of cleaning the lower intestines. Like an enema, it involves taking water into the bowels. Sitting in a tub of water, you insert a round-edged, 4-inch tube into the rectum, then draw the water up by performing Uddiyana Bandha and Nauli. After removing the tube, you use Nauli to churn the water around, then expel it. Whereas enemas force water into the body, in Basti you create a vacuum so that the water is naturally drawn up.

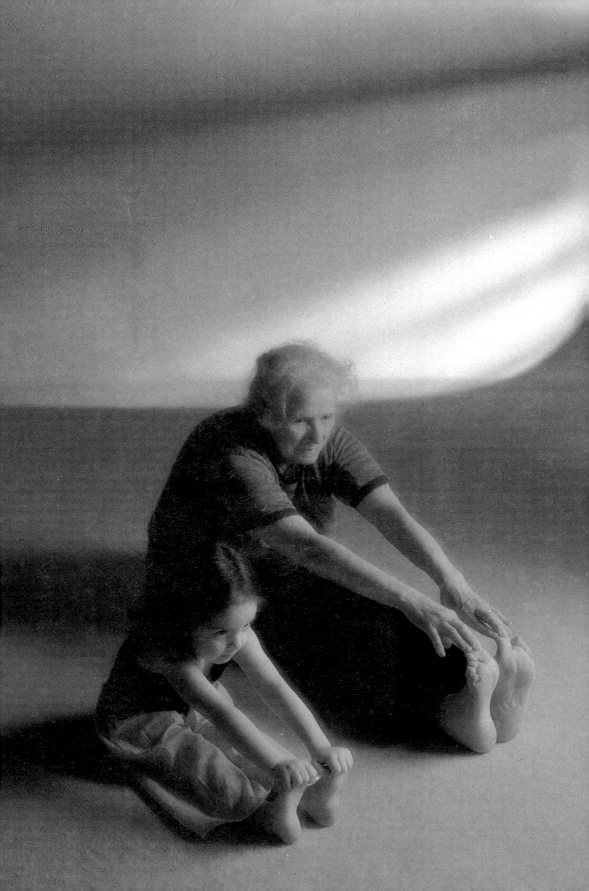

The Cycle of Life

"There is a Spirit which is pure
and which is beyond old age and
death . . . This is Atman, the
Spirit in man."
Chandogya Upanishad

The discipline of yoga provides guidance for a lifetime. It is a versatile and all-embracing science, one that can be modified to suit all stages and conditions of life. You may be drawn initially to the asanas, as a means of staying fit or slim, then discover the value of the breathing exercises or meditation when you enter a time of change. In this section we look at ways of adapting the asanas to suit a variety of needs. We have singled out three periods of life for special attention – Maternity, Childhood and the Later Years. But even if none of these categories relates to your present situation, you can still gain ideas from the material here of how to proceed from your own starting point, always referring to the Basic Session as your foundation for this sequence of asanas.

The serenity of mind that yoga engenders and the physical vitality and suppleness it creates are fundamental to young and old alike. For children it offers a way of maintaining good health throughout life. With their natural resilience and sense of balance, the asanas come easily to them, making the sessions both rewarding and enjoyable. Teenagers too will find enormous benefit in all aspects of practice. Any feelings of self-consciousness or gawkiness will soon be replaced by a new sense of confidence and poise. The techniques of pranayama and relaxation are especially effective in helping to handle the emotional problems that are part and parcel of growing up.

Many women come to yoga when carrying their first child, looking for a way to keep as strong and healthy as possible in pregnancy. The creation of a new life is one of the greatest miracles there are, setting in motion a train of events that will continue for the next seventy or eighty years, and after. There can be no more important time to take care of yourself physically, mentally and spiritually. If you and your partner can establish a good routine of asanas, pranayama and meditation, it will carry you more smoothly through the following periods, the busy early months of caring for a new baby.

The slow gentle movements of the asanas are ideal for the later years of life, helping both mind and body to stay young and active, while the breathing exercises increase the supply of oxygen to the brain. Many asanas can be practised sitting on a chair and some done in the bed. Even if for some reason you are not able to perform the asanas physically, you can try visualizing yourself practising them. This is a tremendous exercise in concentration – but it brings with it many of the benefits that physical practice imparts. The most minute movement can become an asana, when done with awareness and attention to breathing. One yoga student with multiple sclerosis spent several sessions working on bringing her hands together in the prayer pose – for her this was certainly an asana, and one she took great delight in practising and perfecting.

All of us go through times of stress in our lives – whether the cause is a change of job, the break-up of a relationship, or giving up smoking. At these times the regular practice of yoga can provide a port in a storm, giving you the security and sense of continuity you need. Many of our tensions and fears spring from a basic misconception of who we really are. Only when you learn to identify with the Self which is changeless and immortal, will you be able to face the vicissitudes of life with serenity and equanimity.

Maternity

The months of carrying a child are precious, and soon past. A first pregnancy, particularly, is a voyage of discovery, a time of great changes. You are engaged in the creation of a new life, not merely with your body, but with your emotions, mind and spirit too. Yoga will help you to have the best possible pregnancy and delivery, whatever your health or circum-stances, and provide a positive environment for the growing child, right from the start. You will be better able to avoid problems such as overweight, stretch marks and backache. In this section we show you how to amend your asanas, as and when necessary, and introduce special poses for pregnancy and exercises to prepare for an easy delivery. (Read the entire section, including Later Years, as you may find some useful tips there too.) Even if you have never done any yoga before, you will find that practising the simplest poses improves your fitness and well-being, while the relaxation, breathing and meditation help you to handle the whole process, from conception to birth and afterward, with greater assurance and calm. All women experience some fear of labour – but that is just what it is – labour, hard work. Yoga teaches you to face it squarely, to live in the present, taking each event as it comes. Your practice will not only contribute to an easier labour, but also help you to handle any eventuality calmly, from deep resources of strength and energy. Meditation can be very important during pregnancy – study the movement of the mind, turn the mind within, and you will be free of all fears or discomforts. Especially with a first child, it is very important to establish a routine with your asana practice, pranayama and meditation – after the baby arrives the habit will stand you in good stead, carrying you through times of stress and fatigue. Yoga will be a source of strength, helping you to be a more loving, giving mother.

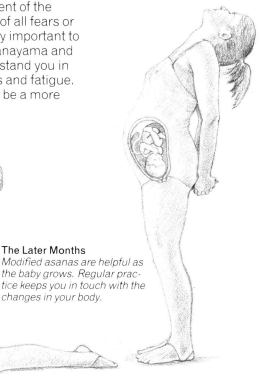

Meditation
Pregnancy is an excellent time for meditation – the way you are feeling and thinking will affect the baby too. As part of your meditation, consciously send prana to the baby in the womb.

Early Pregnancy
Imagine the baby moving with you while you practise asanas.

The Later Months
Modified asanas are helpful as the baby grows. Regular prac-tice keeps you in touch with the changes in your body.

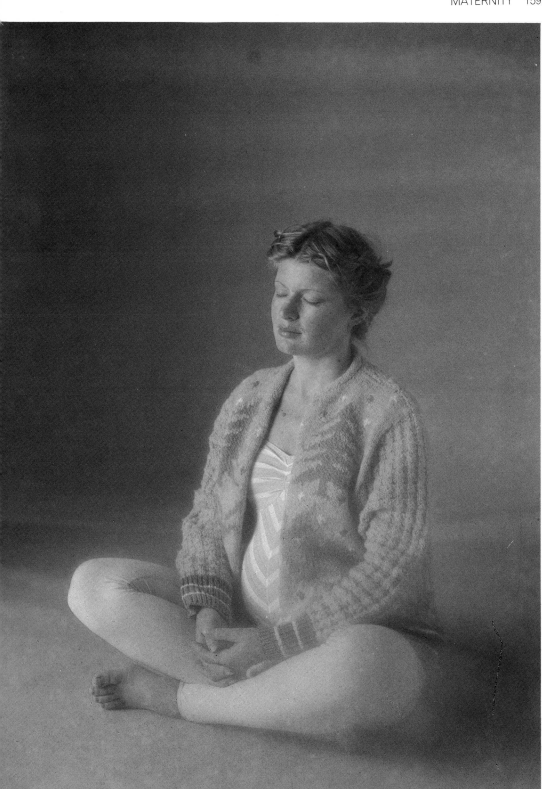

Practice Schedule

This schedule covers the same practice sequence as the Basic Session (pp.30-31), with suggestions for modified asanas and new poses especially suitable during pregnancy. Use it in conjunction with the teaching in the Basic Session, and refer to the charts on pages 54-55 if you want to use a shorter session or need a beginner's programme. If you are already an experienced yoga student, you should keep up a gentle "maintenance" practice during your pregnancy. Your body secretes a hormone called "relaxin" at this time so you may even notice an overall improvement in your asanas. No matter how big you get, you can continue to work on your sitting poses, particularly the Lotus. These sitting poses are very important asanas for you, as they help to open up the pelvis for the birth. So are standing positions, as they strengthen the legs, helping to carry the baby. Because the three basic backward bends – the Locust, Cobra and Bow – are performed on the abdomen, we have suggested alternatives. Listen to your body – you are the best judge of what you can and can't do while you are pregnant and of how to adapt your asanas to meet your own particular needs. Always come out of an asana if you feel any strain or discomfort. But don't be too easy on yourself – the baby is well protected, both by your abdominal muscles and by its sac of amniotic fluid in the womb.

Beginning the Session Start as usual with a few minutes relaxation. If you begin to find the Corpse Pose uncomfortable, try the modified poses on page 169. As the baby grows, come out of any lying down position by rolling to one side and using your hands to push yourself up. **Pranayama** is important – it brings prana to you and the baby, increases your intake of oxygen, and steadies the mind. In labour, if you focus on the breath, it will help you to stay calm, relaxed, and in control.

When doing the **Sun Salutation**, you may have to modify some of the positions slightly, particularly in later months as your abdomen enlarges. Look back to pages 34-35 to refresh your memory of the twelve positions in the sequence.

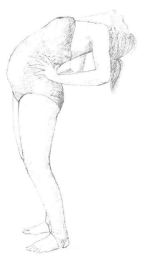

In positions 2 and 11 (backward bending), you can place your hands on your hips, instead of raising them, and spread your feet apart a bit to bring the stretch lower down the back. Between positions 6 and 7, where your abdomen normally brushes against the floor, use your hands to take more of your weight and "ride" from one pose to the next. Feel the baby lying cradled within you.

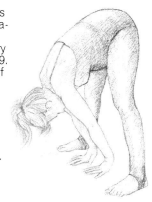

In positions 3 and 10 (forward bending), shown above, there is little problem provided that you spread your legs apart to accommodate the baby.

You should only do Single Leg Raising for these few months, alternating the legs (p.36). You can also try the adapted version in Later Years (p.174). Avoid Double Leg Raising as it puts strain on the abdomen.

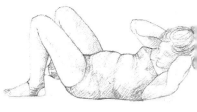

Instead practise the **Pregnancy Sit-up** which will keep the abdominal muscles strong without strain. These muscles, when they are correctly exercised, help to hold the baby correctly in position, so that you are both comfortable. Lie on your back, feet flat on the floor close to your buttocks, and clasp your hands behind your neck. Inhale, lift up the head and shoulders, and twist to the left. Exhale as you go down. Repeat, twisting to the right side. You should do this exercise about five times on each side, feeling how the muscles firm up and hold as you gently raise your head and shoulders then relax gradually downward.

The Headstand and Shoulderstand are invaluable during pregnancy as they rest the lower back, the veins and muscles of the legs, and the muscles of the lower abdomen. They also help to ensure that the womb reverts to its proper position after the birth. However, after the early weeks, getting into and holding these poses may be a little awkward, and your sense of balance may also change. Even if you are proficient at these asanas, you should practise them one step at a time, and stop at once if you feel at all uncertain about going further. If you are a beginner, study the Headstand (p.38) to familiarize yourself with its eight steps, and practise steps 1, 2 and 3 (the "tripod") to gain some of the benefits. Once position 3 is comfortable, you can try lifting up into 4, and walking into 5. You can then modify step 6, by bending and lifting one knee at a time and hold this pose, keeping your spine as straight as possible and breathing deeply.

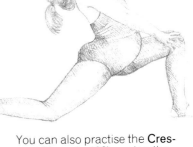

This **Half Headstand** (above) gives most of the benefits of the Headstand pose. Don't attempt to go any further unless you are very proficient. However, if you feel ready, you can try the full pose, practising against a wall for support, but *only in early pregnancy*. Kneeling down with your buttocks close to the wall, make your "tripod", elbows touching knees, and walk in (positions 4 and 5). Then, at 6, walk your feet up the wall, slowly and surely, stopping whenever

you feel the need, till the legs are straight. You can then try lifting first one leg, then the other, away from the wall, until you are able to balance standing free. Keeping close to the wall gives you more confidence, relieving any fears of toppling over. Walk your feet back down the wall to come out of the position.

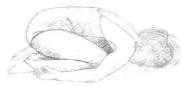

After a full or modified Headstand rest in the **Child's Pose** (p.39), or the modified version with knees spread (as above and p. 169) and breathe deeply until circulation is normal.

For the Shoulderstand and Plough you can use the modified positions on page 164 in this section. If you are a beginner, try simply lying with your feet propped up against a wall. After the Plough, you can add the Wall Stretches. Practise the Fish normally. It is particularly beneficial in helping to combat depression. Push up into the Bridge from the floor – coming from the Shoulderstand is too much abdominal work.

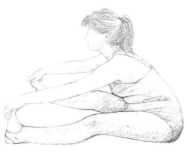

In the **Forward Bend**, take care to accommodate the baby by spreading your thighs apart. As your abdomen grows, you may find the Head to Knee Pose (p.118) more comfortable. The

main point when practising forward bends is to keep the spine straight – when pregnant, your abdomen can serve as a reminder to straighten the back.

The biggest change in your asana session will be with the backward bends. You may find that the three basic ones, the Cobra, Locust and Bow (pp. 50-55), put too much pressure on the abdomen. If so, substitute the Modified Cobra and the Cat (pp. 166-7), and replace the Bow with the Kneeling Wheel (p.130).

You can also practise the **Crescent Moon** (p.132) – using the modified position above, with the hands on the knee for extra support, if this feels better.

The sitting positions should make up a large part of your asanas in pregnancy, as they open up the pelvic area, to give an easier labour, and to strengthen the legs and lower spine. You may even find that your Butterfly and Lotus (p.58) improve, because the pelvic girdle stretches during pregnancy to facilitate the birth. You can also try kneeling poses such as the Warrior (p.130), and Squatting (p.169), to promote elasticity in the vaginal muscles. If you find the Half or full Spinal Twist (pp. 56, 134) put too much pressure on the abdomen, lean back a little to give yourself more space. This is easiest using the version shown on page 174.

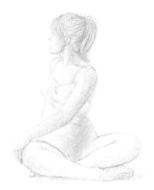

of the front leg. Look toward the back arm. Reverse legs and repeat the twist the other way. Standing positions are useful, as they strengthen the legs, enabling you to carry the child well and to push strongly during labour. Try some of the standing pose variations and asanas shown in the Balancing Cycle on pages 151-152, and practise the Eagle (p.146) – a wonderful exercise to improve circulation and help prevent varicose veins.

Practical matters

During your session, always stop if you feel any strain, and rest frequently in one of the relaxation poses. At the end, relax in the Corpse Pose or a modified version (p.169), for at least ten minutes, preferably longer. As your pregnancy develops, regular asana practice will keep you in touch with the changes in your body, and the growth of the child. You should try to attend a yoga class as often as possible. Rest and deep breathing become more and more important. You should extend your initial and final relaxation periods in a session, and incorporate times to relax into your daily routine. In your Final Relaxation you should practise the sequence on pages 26-27, contracting and relaxing the muscles of different parts of the body in turn and incorporate the Perineal Exercises on page 169. These exercises will gradually teach you to recognize which particular muscles are tense, and then relax them consciously. During labour you will be able to relax between contractions, and so avoid becoming tired.

Alternatively, sit cross-legged in the **Easy Pose** for a modified twist. Place your left hand on the outside of your right knee for leverage, and your right hand on the floor behind you, and twist gently to the right. Look to the right. Hold the position, and breathe deeply. Repeat on the other side.

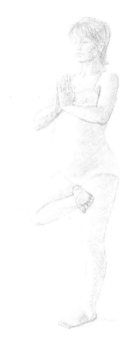

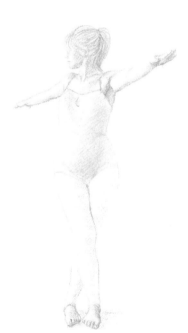

The **Standing Spinal Twist** (above) puts no pressure on the abdomen. Cross your legs, stretch your arms out to the sides, and twist in the direction

The **Tree** (above) has similar benefits, and also – like all balancing asanas – helps to improve your concentration and steady your mind. The calming influence of the asanas will be enormously rewarding during the months to come. Practice the steps into the Tree first, as described on page 146, placing your foot high against the opposite thigh. If you find this easy, try it with the raised leg in the Half Lotus, as illustrated. Soon you will be able to hold the pose with eyes closed.

The Scorpion
Yoga students with many years' experience develop a sureness that permits them to carry on doing advanced poses like the Scorpion (right) throughout pregnancy. This photograph is intended to inspire you, to show you just what the pregnant body is capable of achieving.

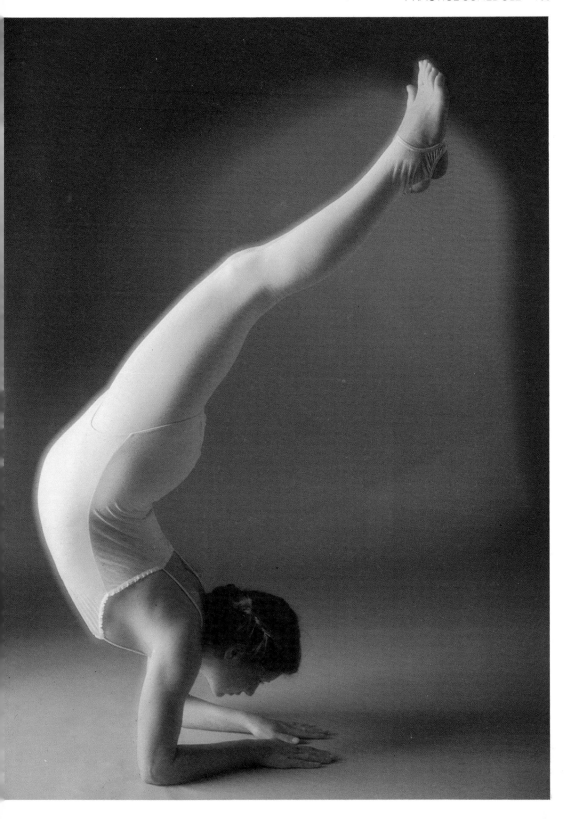

Special Asanas for Pregnancy

As the baby grows, you may begin to feel a little cumbersome, and find it harder to practise some of the most useful asanas in the normal way. You can replace the basic inverted poses, which strengthen the back and rest the heart and legs, with the positions shown here (and on p. 161). Instead of your usual backward bends, practise the Cat and the Modified Cobra, which help to prevent a sagging abdomen and stretch-marks, and strengthen the legs, so that you can carry the child well. During these months you will also be preparing your body for the birth – the Wall Stretches and Squatting Pose will open up the pelvis, and the Perineal Exercises tone the pelvic and vaginal muscles. Lastly, try the amended Corpse Poses if you need them, to relax, and sleep, comfortably.

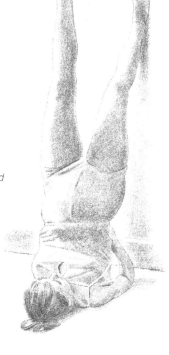

Modified Shoulderstand

The Shoulderstand is most refreshing and invigorating – especially in pregnancy when extra weight makes your legs and back tired. But if your expanding tummy makes it harder to get into the position, use a wall for support and reassurance, pressing with your feet to take some of the weight as you walk up. You will be obtaining all the benefits of inverting your body without the effort of supporting your full body weight.

Modified Shoulderstand
Lie with buttocks against the wall, legs stretched up it. Press on your feet, lifting yourself enough to insert your hands and support your back (p. 40). Walk up until your legs are straight, then practise lifting one leg at a time (or both legs) off the wall.

Modified Plough
From the modified Shoulder-stand, bring one or both legs over to rest on a chair behind you, pushing your heels back.

Modified Plough

For greater comfort in the Plough you can separate your legs. Or, if your feet don't reach the floor, use a chair to take some of your weight. Pressing your feet into a chair has the added benefit of improving your stretch. This technique is useful for beginners too, before the full Plough is achieved.

Caution Make sure the chair cannot possibly move.

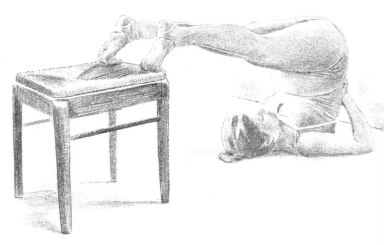

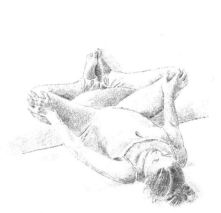

Wall Squatting
Separate your feet widely and place the soles flat on the wall. Gently pull your knees out and down with your hands, press ing your feet against the wall. As a variation, try doing the Side Splits against the wall.

Wall Stretches

These positions are restful and refreshing, and gently open up your pelvis for the birth. Lying on the floor keeps your spine straight – often a problem in leg stretches from a sitting position. And with the floor and wall taking your weight, you can put all your energy into the stretch. You can also perform these stretches passively, arms re- laxed along the floor.

Wall Butterfly
Lie with your buttocks and feet against the wall, soles together, and let your knees drop open. Use your hands to press your knees down and toward the wall. Rest and enjoy the pose.

The Pelvic Lift

This exercise strengthens the uterus, the muscular cradle for the growing child, and also en- courages deep breathing and eases lower back strain. The "all fours" position makes you feel strong and healthy – and some mothers find it comfortable dur- ing labour. The Pelvic Lift both stretches and counterstretches the entire spine.

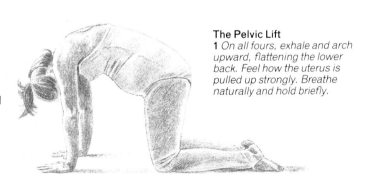

The Pelvic Lift
1 *On all fours, exhale and arch upward, flattening the lower back. Feel how the uterus is pulled up strongly. Breathe naturally and hold briefly.*

2 *Inhale, and arch downward, curving the lower back. Lift your head up and back and breathe naturally. Repeat 1 and 2 slowly, several times.*

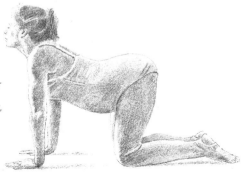

Modified Cobra

This pose is more suitable than the classic Cobra (p.50) during pregnancy, as it avoids abdominal pressure and strengthens the legs while still giving a good backward bend. It consists of three stages, lowering the bend from the cervical, through thoracic to lumbar vertebrae. Practise one step at a time at first – hold each stage, breathing normally and stretch further only when you feel ready. Soon you will be able to combine the stages into a flowing movement. Keeping the feet together gives the best stretch, but you can separate them for comfort.

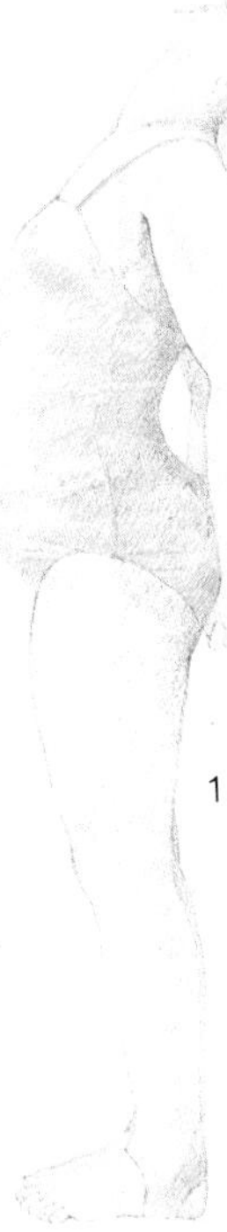

1

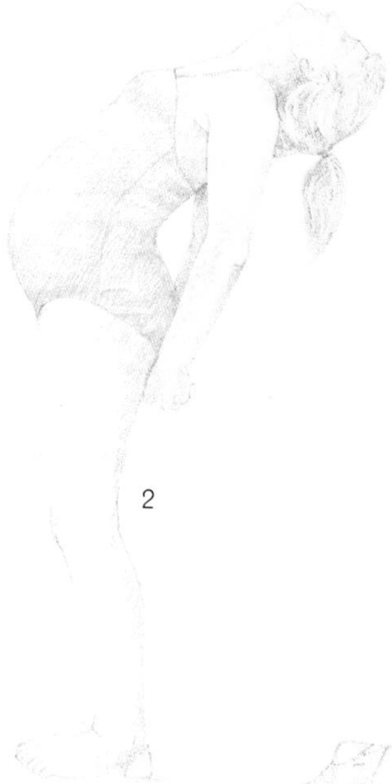

2

Modified Cobra
Stand with feet together, and hands clasped behind back.
1 Inhale and drop the head back. Hold and breathe gently.
2 Inhale and arch back, pushing your chest out and arms back.
3 (far right) Inhale and push your hips forward, your arms right back. Rest in the Child's Pose.

The Cat

Performed comfortably on all fours, without any strain on the abdomen, this asana serves to replace the Locust (p.52) in your practice during pregnancy. The pose keeps the lower back limber and strengthens the legs. As well as the movements shown here, try bringing the knee of the raised leg in to the forehead at the end, as a counterpose.

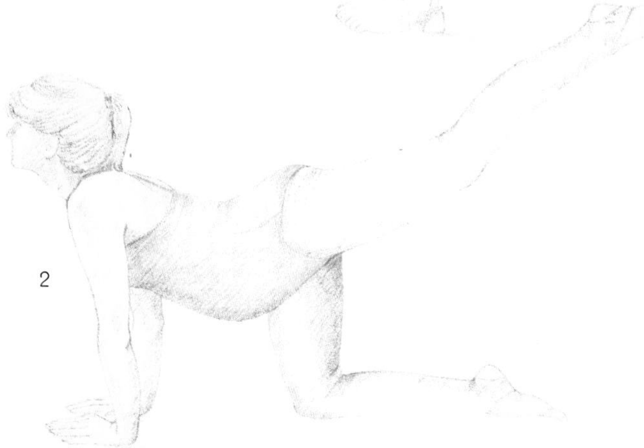

2

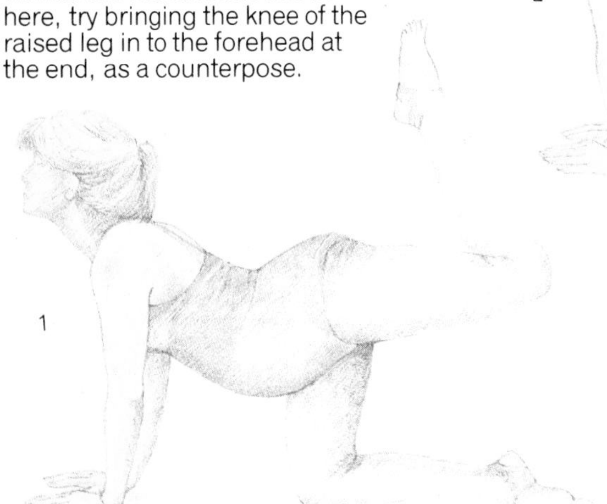

1

The Cat
1 Kneeling on all fours, inhale and lift one leg straight up behind you, raising your head at the same time. Hold the pose, breathing normally, then exhale and lower the leg. Change legs.
2 Proceed as above, but bend the raised leg and point the toes toward your head. When you are ready, perform both steps in one.

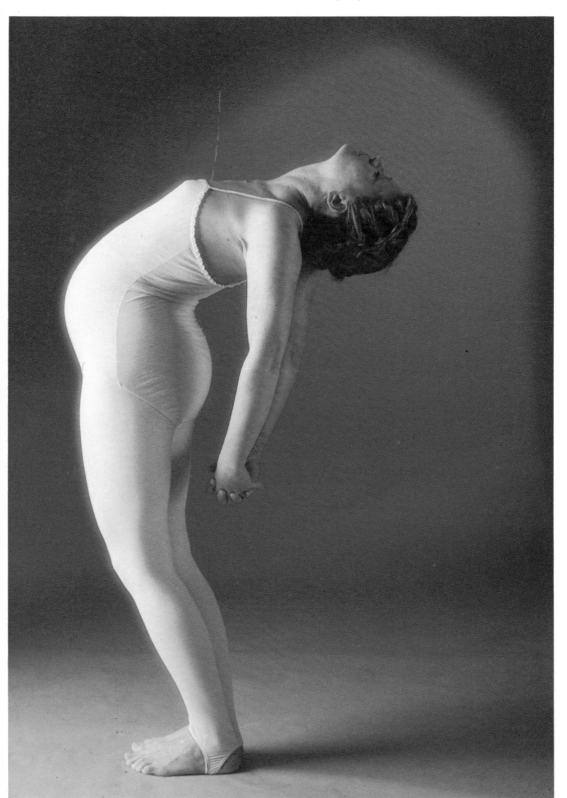

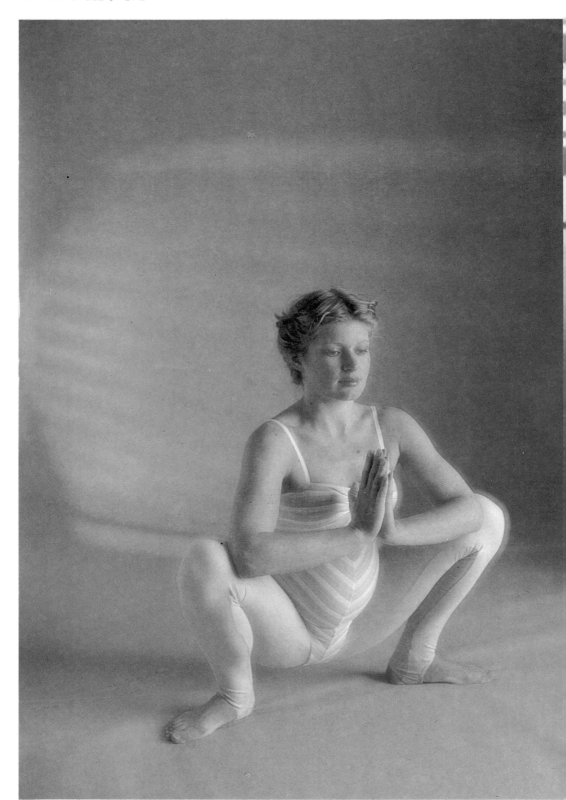

Perineal Exercises

These exercises keep the pelvic, anal and vaginal muscles strong and healthy. Like good elastic, they will stretch fully for the birth and quickly return to normal, avoiding postnatal problems like a prolapse or a leaky bladder. They also help you to develop awareness and control of the muscles, so that you can actively help in an easier birth.

Exercise 1 Lie comfortably on your back, ankles crossed. Tilt the pelvis up, pressing the small of your back against the floor. Exhale, squeeze your thighs together, and clench the buttocks, contracting the pelvic muscles. Hold for a count of five, inhale, and relax.

Exercise 2 (Aswini Mudra) Sit, squat or stand comfortably. Exhale, and contract the muscles of the anal sphincter. Hold for a count of five, inhale, and relax. Exhale again, and contract the vaginal muscles. Hold for five, inhale, and relax.

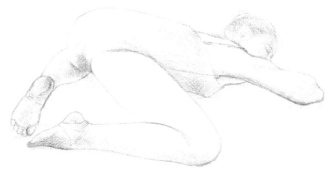

Modified Child's Pose
You can adapt the Child's Pose (p.39) simply by spreading the knees wide apart to accommodate the abdomen.

Relaxation

Especially during the last few months of pregnancy – just when rest is most important – it can be difficult to find comfortable positions for relaxation and sleeping. The two poses shown here provide useful alternatives. The Modified Child's Pose (above) not only gives you a comfortable resting posture and a gentle forward bend, but also helps to open the pelvic area. Raising one knee while lying on your front (below) supports the weight of the abdomen and makes breathing easier. By alternating which leg is bent, you gently stretch and compress each side of the body in turn, like a mini asana. You can also experiment with using pillows to make yourself more comfortable – try lying on your side with a pillow between your knees, for example, to ease strain on the pelvis and lower back.

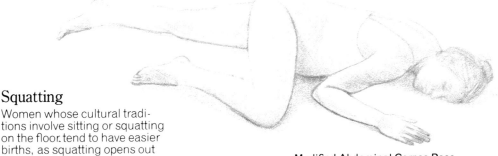

Squatting

Women whose cultural traditions involve sitting or squatting on the floor tend to have easier births, as squatting opens out the pelvic area and strengthens the legs. It also keeps the lower back supple and provides gentle abdominal pressure, ensuring good circulation and preventing constipation. If you are not used to squatting, use a chair to support yourself.

Squatting Pose (left)
Use a chair for support at first, and squat on your toes. Your heels will gradually come down.

Modified Abdominal Corpse Pose
This pose may be more comfortable in later pregnancy, as it helps to take the weight of the baby off the abdomen and distribute it over the rest of the body. Support your head on one or both arms – whichever you find easier for breathing – and alternate which leg is drawn up.

Childhood

Starting yoga when young gives children the best foundation in life. With their natural flexibility and sense of balance, they usually find it far easier to adopt the postures than adults, and can make rapid progress. The majority of children are naturally adventurous – all they need is a little encouragement. Help them to get into the correct position, but take care never to force their bodies into a pose, as bones and muscles are still growing. Most children are great mimics – if they see you practising your asanas regularly they will want to join in and imitate what you do. Generally, the only problem is one of concentration, as a child's attention span is not normally very long. The solution, especially with a young child, is to stimulate their interest by making the sessions fun. Make use

Yoga for the Young
The children in these pictures range from two to eleven. Shown below are the Wheel (top left); Easy Pose and Lotus (top right); Half Locust and Camel (bottom left); Cobra (bottom centre); Eagle (bottom right) and Corpse Pose (far right).

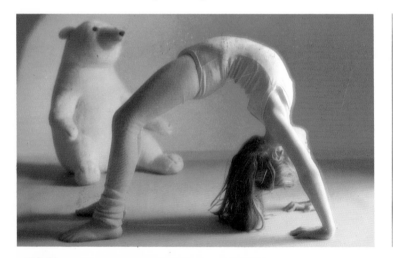

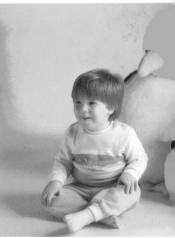

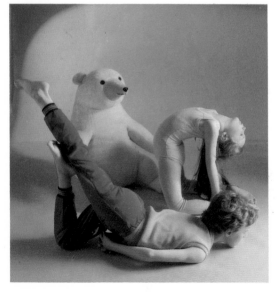

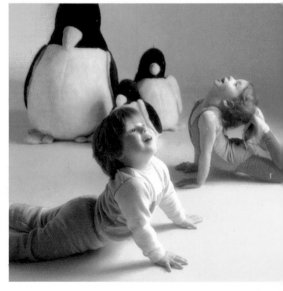

of the fact that many asanas are named after animals, birds and other creatures – let the child roar like a lion or arch up like a snake-charmer's cobra. Use your imagination – practising the Forward Bend is like closing a book, the Shoulderstand is like the candle on a birthday cake. It is also most important to learn how to breathe correctly at a young age. Try teaching a small child abdominal breathing in the Corpse Pose – place a rubber duck on his tummy and let him see how the duck swims as he breathes gently in and out. Meditation too is of great value when growing up, strengthening a child's powers of concentration. In schools where meditation is taught, teachers have observed a great improvement both in class work and in group interaction.

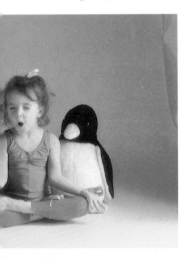

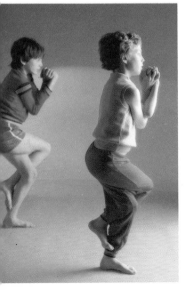

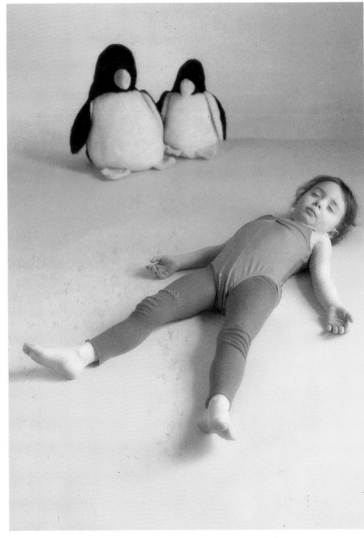

The Later Years

It's never too late to take up yoga, whether you are five or a hundred and five – you are only as old as you feel. The later years of life can truly be golden – you have time to devote to yourself both physically and spiritually. Many of the problems of later life are compounded by insufficient exercise, unwise eating habits and shallow breathing – problems such as poor circulation, arthritis and digestive disorders. But your body has incredible regenerative powers and even after a short time of practising yoga you will sleep better and have more energy and a more positive approach to life. If you have been inactive for some time, take the asanas slowly and gently at first. Start with the exercises shown opposite. Then go on to include some of the asanas from the Basic Session, gradually incorporating more until you have learned them all. You will benefit far more from peaceful movements that you enjoy than from vigorous exercises you find a strain. If some of the postures seem a little advanced, modify them to begin with to suit your abilities – a few examples are shown on page 174. Be kind to yourself and patient with your body's shortcomings. Try not to extend yourself to the point where you get out of breath – but if this happens, simply relax in the Corpse Pose until your breathing has returned to normal. At the same time, don't be over-indulgent, limiting yourself by expecting too little of your body. After a few months' practise you will be surprised to discover that you can do things you never believed possible. If you find that you are too stiff to do your asanas in the morning, have a hot bath first or practise them in the afternoon, when your body has had a chance to loosen up. Be sure to practise pranayama and meditation every day. Proper breathing is of great importance in later life (see p.68) and meditation will help you to feel centered in your self and diminish fear and loneliness. Realise that this body is just a vehicle for the soul – the real Self is immortal.

Sivananda's Pranayama
This simple breathing exercise stills the mind, helps the circulation and brings a feeling of peace and harmony. You can include it in your daily pranayama using the sitting pose of your choice, or even practise it in bed. Breathe in through both nostrils, slowly retain the breath, then breathe out fully. Make the inhalation, retention and exhalation as long as you find comfortable. Practise ten rounds.

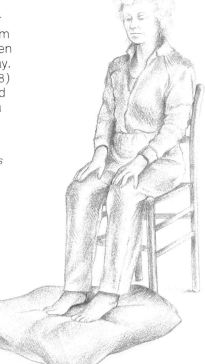

Modified Sitting Poses
Sit in one of the meditative poses – with a pillow under your buttocks, or sit on a chair, spine erect. Put a pillow under your feet – don't let them dangle.

Warm-Up Exercises

You can use these movements either to prepare you for your Basic Session of asanas or as a self-contained sequence, until you are ready to begin the asanas. The idea is to move every part of your body, easing any stiffness in the joints and improving circulation, especially to the extremities. You can perform exercises 1, 3, 4 and 5 from either a standing position or sitting down. Try to integrate your breathing and make your movements gentle. Repeat each exercise several times.

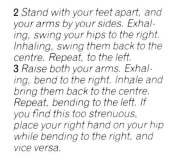

2 *Stand with your feet apart, and your arms by your sides. Exhaling, swing your hips to the right. Inhaling, swing them back to the centre. Repeat, to the left.*
3 *Raise both your arms. Exhaling, bend to the right. Inhale and bring them back to the centre. Repeat, bending to the left. If you find this too strenuous, place your right hand on your hip while bending to the right, and vice versa.*

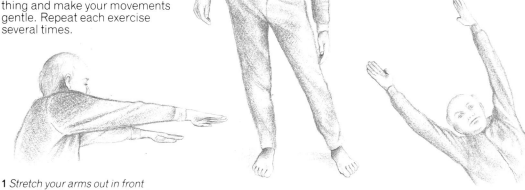

1 *Stretch your arms out in front of you. Exhaling, twist head and body to the right. Inhaling, twist back to the centre. Exhaling, twist to the left. Inhaling, twist back to the centre.*

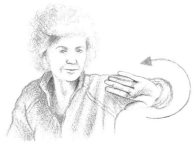
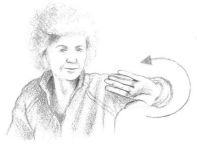

5 *One at a time, rotate your arms from the shoulder, first backward and then forward. Now rotate each forearm from the elbow, backward and forward.*

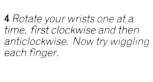

4 *Rotate your wrists one at a time, first clockwise and then anticlockwise. Now try wiggling each finger.*

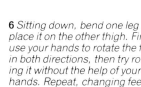
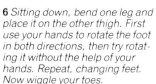

6 *Sitting down, bend one leg and place it on the other thigh. First use your hands to rotate the foot in both directions, then try rotating it without the help of your hands. Repeat, changing feet. Now wiggle your toes.*

Modified Asanas

If you are just beginning yoga, you may prefer to approach the Basic Session gently. Here are a few examples of how you can modify the basic asanas; additional ideas are to be found in the Maternity section (pp. 160-169). Have a suitable chair and a nice plump pillow ready before you start practising. Use these props to assist you but not to force your body further than is comfortable. When practising asanas, always make sure that you are warm enough.

Basic Asanas *(right)*
The Headstand (top left), the Shoulderstand (top right) and the Plough (below).

Single Leg Raising
Keep one leg bent, foot flat on the floor, while you raise the other leg. This will demand less effort from the abdominal and lower back muscles.

Backward Bending *(above)*
Using a pillow you can develop flexibility without strain. Lean back on your elbows, lower your head to the floor. Try it with legs straight, then kneel and stretch your arms back.

Half Spinal Twist
With your lower leg straight, it is easier to balance. If necessary, lean back a little as you twist to each side.

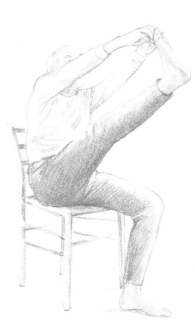

Forward Bending
You can obtain many of the benefits of the Forward Bend while sitting in a chair. Perform this modified asana in two stages. First, fold forward, keeping your back as straight as possible, and place your hands on the floor by your feet, as shown left. Then, to stretch your hamstrings, hold one foot and pull the leg up as high as you can, as shown right. The other leg balances you.

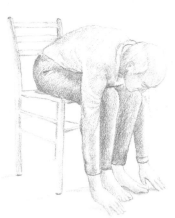

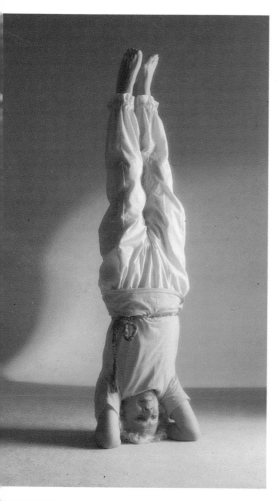

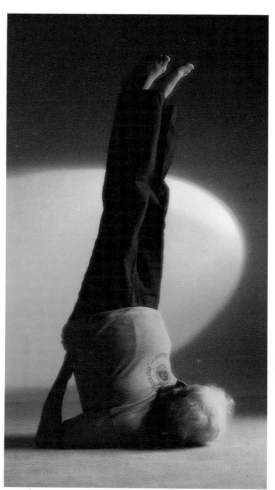

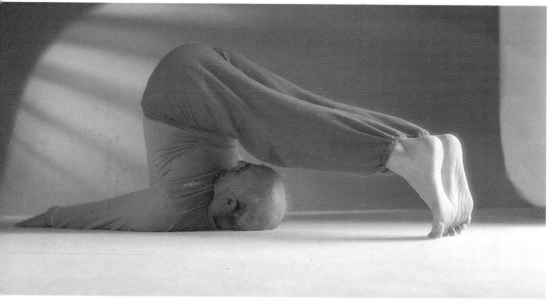

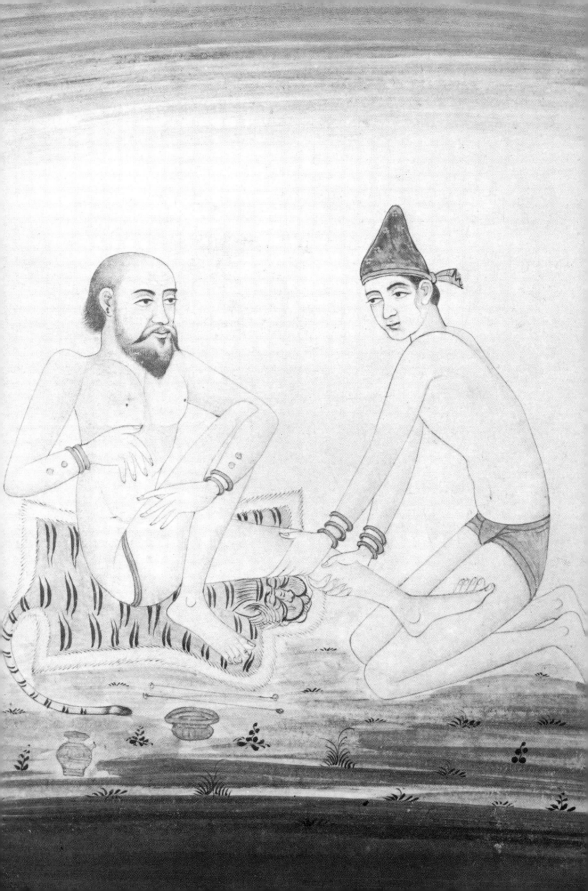

Yoga and Health

"The Yogi regards the physical body
as an instrument for his journey
toward perfection."
Swami Vishnu Devananda

Yoga is a science of health – unlike modern Western medicine which is largely a science of disease and treatment. The teachings of yoga are based on an intricate and precise understanding of the healthy functioning of the human body and mind, and its techniques are designed to maximise your own potential for good health, vitality and lasting youthfulness. When you practise yoga in your daily life, you are like a car owner who maintains and services his own vehicle, keeping it running in tip top condition and gleaming like new, year in, year out. Without this discipline, you are like a car owner whose vehicle will not start in the morning, needs expensive servicing and occasional major repairs, and may ultimately break down at a critical moment, with serious consequences.

The natural state of the body is health – every smallest part and function has one overriding biological aim, to seek and restore health at all times. Wounds heal, bones mend, fevers abate, toxins are removed, fatigue is repaired – we have at our command a miracle of bio-engineering which should last us into a peaceful and healthy later life.

This section describes the functioning of this remarkable living system, looking in particular at three major functions: the body's strong, flexible frame of muscles, bones and ligaments; the nutrient cycles of digestion, respiration and circulation which nourish and service every cell and tissue; and the vital messenger systems of nerves and hormones which balance and regulate our physical, emotional and mental responses. Yoga, unique among all forms of bodily culture, works systematically on all these parts of the living body to keep them functioning in balance and in perfect condition.

In contemporary life, the experience of full and vital health is a rarity after childhood. Taking our bodies for granted, we abuse them without thought. We spend long hours shut off from air and sunlight, sitting uncomfortably, snatching hurriedly cooked meals, finding no time to stretch our bodies, allow them free movement, deeper relaxation, clean air, or fresh, natural foods. If our bodies complain, we take pills – silencing the very signals that might alert us to trouble, and further damaging the body's natural repair systems. By getting these natural systems working in balance again, yoga can do much to restore good health even after years of unhealthy living have resulted in the ailments familiar to us all – stress, fatigue, hypertension, insomnia, rheumatism, and so on.

Much of the illness and loss of vitality we suffer arises from long-term running down of the body systems, due to under-use and under-stimulation of vital functions. Exercise is now advocated by all health disciplines, but the yoga exercises are unique. The principle yogis have understood for thousands of years is that proper exercise is designed, not to develop muscle and exhaust our strength, but to gently stretch and tone the body and above all to stimulate circulation, right down to the cellular level, so that tissues are nourished, wastes removed, vital organs returned to full efficiency, and the metabolism of health is restored.

The physical body is only one aspect of health in yoga philosophy – mind and spirit are just as important. Western medicine too, has begun to understand that the mind must heal, for the body to mend. But the Western approach is piecemeal – whereas yoga integrates the science of mind, body and spirit.

The Body's Frame

The most remarkable feat of balance we perform each day is simply standing upright on two feet. The human frame aligns itself to support and distribute our weight with the greatest economy of effort – the arch of the foot, the precise curves of the spine, the design of every joint, the tilt of the pelvis – and is designed to combine freedom of movement with strength, and protection of the vital organs. The joints are held firmly by strong, elastic ligaments, and the whole structure is supported, moved and returned to alignment by the muscles.

The skeletal muscles work on the principle of a balance of opposing forces – as one muscle contracts to produce movement, another relaxes and stretches to allow it. If the stretching or "antagonistic" muscle is stiff and weak with underuse, the contracting one cannot work efficiently – this is why we stretch and yawn to get our bodies moving. Stress can lead to permanently tensed muscles, which oppose every movement, and make each action doubly tiring. Removing this tension through yoga relaxation techniques gives a rejuvenating ease of movement, and freedom from aches and pains. The process of ageing can also cause the ligaments that bind the joints and the surface of muscles to lose tone and tighten; a sudden strain may then tear or snap them.

Yoga asanas give muscles and ligaments a slow, nonviolent stretch, without the following sharp contraction of most sports. Stretching a muscle helps it to contract more strongly, while the slow movements and deep breathing increase the oxygen supply to the muscles, preventing the accumulation of lactic acid in the fibres. The stretching and contracting muscles stimulate circulation to the tissues and organs, and cause an increased venous return.

As children, we delight in exercising every smallest muscle. This natural activity keeps the body fit and the musculature balanced. But as adults, our range of movements is limited by repetitive tasks. Long hours of sitting at a desk, head thrust forward and lower spine rounded, can cause the ligaments at the base of the skull to shorten, so that trying to straighten up produces pain, sometimes all down the spine (as the spinal ligaments are interconnected) – the Fish and Shoulderstand are helpful after a day of desk work. Poor posture generally leads to undue stress on the lower spine and the hips and pelvis, with back ache and stiffness resulting. Even such a simple action as carrying a bag always on the same shoulder can soon throw the whole frame out, with muscles overdeveloped on one side, until a vertebra may be displaced. The Forward Bend is a good corrective asana here. But for all such common health problems, prevention is better than cure – regular practice of the full asana sequence, which is designed to stimulate the circulation, and to work systematically on every part of the body so that the muscles are healthy and in balance, will keep you young and agile throughout your life.

Muscles

Your skeletal muscles are ranged symmetrically, left to right and front to back, in layers with different actions. Each muscle has an insertion at the pulling point, and an origin at an anchoring point. Muscles usually work in pairs – when your knee bends, for instance, the flexor contracts to pull, the extensor relaxes to allow the bend; when you straighten it, the reverse happens. Similarly, elevators and depressors raise and lower a part; adductors and abductors move it toward or away from the centre line of the body. There are also rotators to pivot a part, tensors to make a joint rigid, sphincters, and some special movements. Yoga asanas systematically work each opposing set of muscles in turn (as for example in the forward and backward bends, below), keeping them youthful, elastic and in balance with each other. The illustrations here give an impression of the principal muscles of the surface layers. (The deep muscles of the spinal column are not visible.)

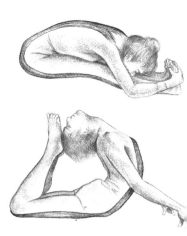

The Head to Knee (top) works the extensors of knee, foot and neck, stretching hamstrings and back muscles. **The Cobra** works the flexors of knee, foot (plantar), spine and neck.

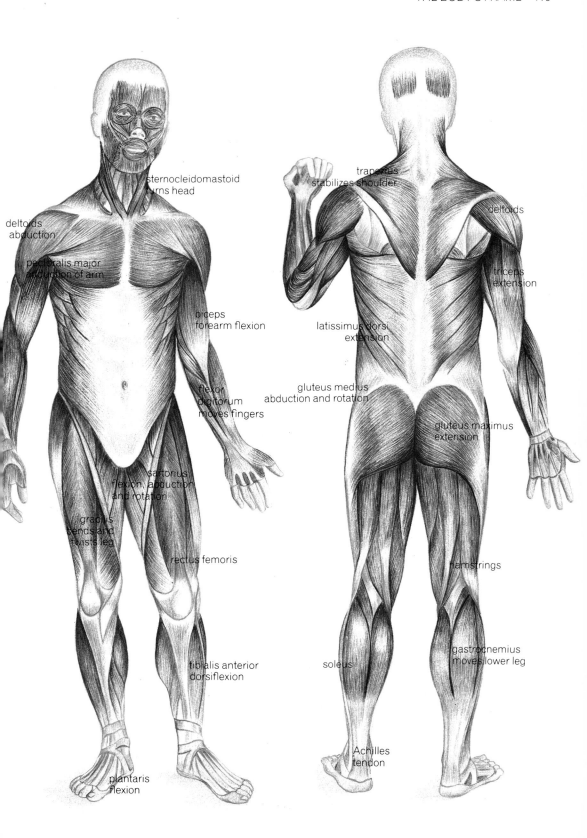

sternocleidomastoid
turns head

deltoids
abduction

pectoralis major
adduction of arm

biceps
forearm flexion

flexor
digitorum
moves fingers

sartorius
flexion, abduction
and rotation

gracilis
bends and
twists leg

rectus femoris

tibialis anterior
dorsiflexion

plantaris
flexion

trapezius
stabilizes shoulder

deltoids

triceps
extension

latissimus dorsi
extension

gluteus medius
abduction and rotation

gluteus maximus
extension

hamstrings

gastrocnemius
moves lower leg

soleus

Achilles
tendon

The Skeleton

Our bodies depend on an intricate framework of some 206 bones. The axial skeleton comprises skull, breastbone, ribs and the column of vertebrae guarding the vital spinal cord. The successive arcs of the spine (cervical, thoracic, lumbar and sacral) give it resilience, and effective weight distribution. Problems of these spinal curves – round shoulders, hollow back, and twisted spine – cause increased stress on lumbar vertebrae, and on the joints of the limbs, pelvis and pectoral girdle. These joints are protected from wear by cartilage, and supported in correct position by muscles and ligaments. Your asanas are designed to free all the body's different joints, opening them up to relieve pressure on the protective cartilage and restore correct alignment of the bones. By keeping muscles and ligaments healthy, and posture correct, you can prevent problems from damage of joints.

Intervertebral discs

Between the vertebrae, pads of cartilage with a soft, gelatinous centre act as buffers, to absorb shock and allow movement. In rest, each disc has a rounded shape, below left; in normal standing positions, the centre of the disc is compressed by the body weight, below right. Strenuous or sudden movement can

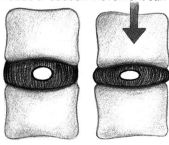

cause a 'slipped disc' – cartilage bulges out, pressing on an adjacent spinal nerve, giving intense pain and immobilising the spine. A yoga teacher could recommend helpful asanas, and you can prevent any recurrence with work to strengthen the spine, and relaxation to rest the discs.

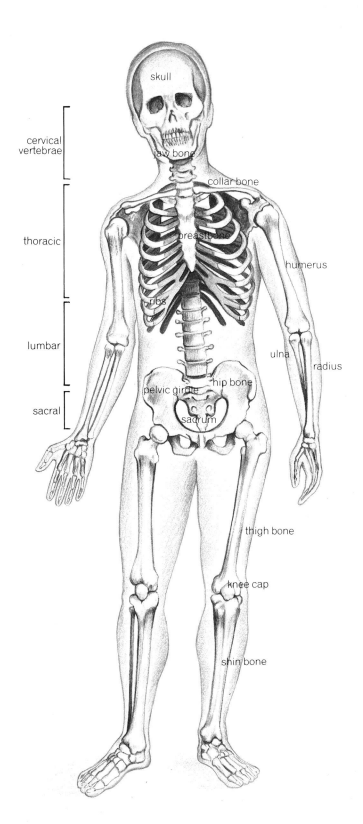

skull

cervical
vertebrae

jaw bone

collar bone

thoracic

breastbone

humerus

ribs

lumbar

ulna

radius

hip bone

pelvic girdle

sacral

sacrum

thigh bone

knee cap

shin bone

Spinal Movements

The body is designed to allow a remarkable range of movements of the limbs and spine. This potential is much underused, partly because we are not aware of it, and more because we allow the ligaments of the joints, spine and muscles to tighten with disuse. The spinal column can be "flexed" or bent forward, "extended" or bent backward, bent sideways, rotated, and swayed or "circumducted" in a combination of movements. The limit of spinal movement is determined by three factors: the knobbed construction of the vertebrae, the length of the spinal ligaments, and the condition of the antagonistic muscles. The asanas shown here illustrate the maximum potential for movement of the healthy spine and pelvis. The flexibility of the spine varies between individuals and with use, so do not be disheartened if you cannot approach the positions shown. All that stands between you and the natural flexibility of your frame is practice.

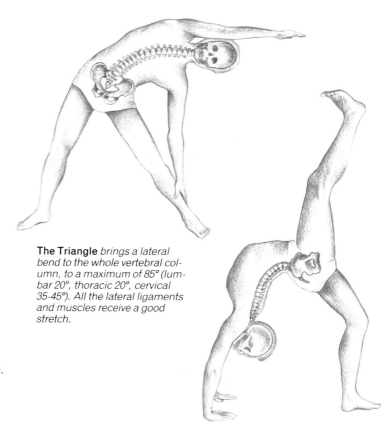

The Triangle *brings a lateral bend to the whole vertebral column, to a maximum of 85° (lumbar 20°, thoracic 20°, cervical 35-45°). All the lateral ligaments and muscles receive a good stretch.*

The Child's Pose *gives the frame a forward bend of 110°. The asana relaxes spinal ligaments, stretches the back muscles, and relieves the compression of the lumbar intervertebral discs normally present when standing.*

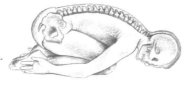

The Wheel Variation *gives the spine its maximum backward bend – a total of 140° (neck 75°, thoraco-lumbar region 65°). The muscles involved are flexors of the back, the supporting leg, and wrists, and extensors of the arms and raised leg.*

The Corpse Pose *removes all stress from the spine, and restores its natural symmetry. The sacrum pushes the pelvis upward, allowing it to open up at the sides under the pull of gravity, resting the intervertebral discs completely.*

The Wind Relieving Pose *tilts the pelvis and flexes the hips, separating the sacroiliac joint. Maximum flexion of the pelvis in this pose is 30°.*

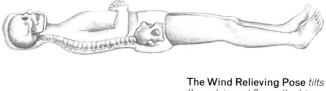

The Nutrient Cycles

The body is the temple of the spirit, and we should care for it as such. Ultimately, the health of your body depends on the health of its living cells, the building blocks of the tissues and organs whose diverse functions are vital to our well being. Cells and tissues need a proper environment for health – free of toxins, rich in the necessary supplies of nutrients, and with an efficient communications system. The urgent need of every cell is to obtain oxygen to fuel its work, and to get rid of waste carbon dioxide quickly. Healthy lungs and heart are the first essential for the cells to obtain the right nutrients. By eating the right food for you, at correct times of day, you will have a healthy digestion, and the blood will absorb and excrete waste – products thoroughly. The micro-circulation around the cells is the body's foundation of health and vitality.

When you press an area of your skin, it turns first paler, as the blood is pushed away, and then red as it rushes back. This is how yoga asanas work on your tissues, like a hand slowly and gently squeezing a sponge to remove all the stale, waste bearing fluids, and then stretching the tissues to allow fresh, life-giving nutrients and energy to circulate to every cell. Breathing deeply as you hold the asana sends more oxygen into the cells, and removes more carbon dioxide. Increased venous return stimulates the heart to contract more firmly in response. The asanas also massage the vital organs, and stimulate the digestive muscles to increase their peristalsis.

The patterns of modern living have a particularly deleterious effect at the tissue level. Sitting still for a long time without moving or stretching the body allows the micro-circulation, and the major circulation too, to grow sluggish. We breathe polluted air, or smoke, and eat foods containing a range of substances that the body cannot use, or are actually toxic. When circulation is sluggish, kidneys and liver are not kept at full efficiency, and toxins build up and clog the tissues. Meat, for instance, contains more uric acid than we normally excrete, and this can damage tissues, and is implicated in gout and rheumatoid arthritis.

Uncomfortable symptoms such as indigestion, varicose veins or headaches are like the warning lights on a car, telling us that the vehicle is about to break down. While specific asanas can alleviate them, treating symptoms and ignoring the proper functioning of your whole system is like disconnecting the car's warning lights, so they will not annoy you. Yoga teaches that you must treat the body as a whole, as every part affects the rest, and be aware of the intimate relationships of body and mind. If you think positively, every cell in your body will be affected. And if you change your pattern of living, founding it instead on the five principles of health (p.21), you will get your whole system working at its best, so that every function of your body operates in a healthier environment.

Digestion

The continuous massaging of the digestive organs by the respiratory movements of the diaphragm helps keep them healthy. Backward and Forward Bends, and the Spinal Twist assist this process. Agni Sara, below, works directly on the diaphragm.

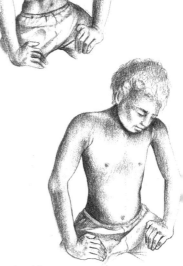

Agni Sara
The pumping action of this asana is particularly useful for the digestion. Take a wide stance, knees bent, hands pressing on thighs, looking down at the abdomen. Exhaling, pull the abdomen in and up, hold the breath, and pump the tummy in and out. When you need to inhale, cease pumping, take a normal breath, exhale and continue. Ten to eighteen pumpings are enough each time.

Respiration

The lungs are the gateway to the body's oxygen supply. Healthy, elastic lungs will expand fully on a deep breath, dilating all the tiny air sacs where the exchange of gases with the blood takes place, and then recoil deeply to expel the waste carbon dioxide (though not completely, as a residue of air always remains in the lungs). Yoga asanas and abdominal breathing improve all your respiratory functions, increasing vital capacity (air intake) and developing strong muscles and elastic tissues, while pranayama teaches breath control and keeps air passages clear. Particularly helpful are the Locust and Peacock, for deep inhalation and breath-holding; Nauli and Uddiyana Bhanda for deep exhalation; and Kapalabhati to exercise the diaphragm.

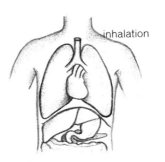

inhalation

exhalation

Respiratory muscles
Your lungs work like bellows, in the partial vacuum of the thoracic cavity. To suck in air, the cavity enlarges – the rib cage expands, and the diaphragm moves down, massaging the abdominal organs. When you exhale, air is expelled as the abdomen contracts, the rib cage recoils and the diaphragm moves up, massaging the heart.

Air passages
The nasal passages filter, warm and moisten the air as it is drawn down to the lungs via the larynx and trachea. This is partly why you breathe through the nose for yoga asanas. If you have a head cold or sore throat, the Shoulderstand, Fish and Lion Pose are helpful.

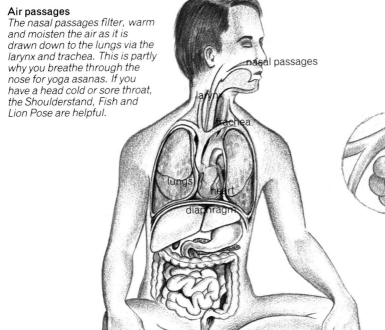

nasal passages

larynx

trachea

lungs

heart

diaphragm

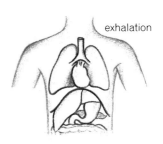

bronchioli

Air sacs
In the lungs, the bronchi divide finely, terminating in the alveoli or air sacs. If your breathing is shallow, the furthest air sacs remain idle, and deteriorate – oxygen intake is reduced and infection is more likely. In allergenic or nervous conditions such as hay fever and asthma, tightening of the small tubes and air sacs of the lungs occurs; relaxation, pranayama and abdominal breathing can be helpful.

Circulation

The blood stream is the body's major transport system, carrying red blood cells to ferry oxygen to the tissues and remove carbon dioxide, white cells to fight infection, nutrients, messenger chemicals, and so on. Efficient circulation depends on a healthy heart, and on elastic and unobstructed blood vessels, from the major arteries and veins to the tiny capillaries. All the asanas are beneficial to circulation, particularly the inverted poses, below. Nauli and Kapalabhati massage the heart, while the alternate increase and decrease in pressure on the heart created by the asana sequence helps to build a stronger heart muscle.

Leg veins and valves
Movement of your leg muscles pushes used blood collected in peripheral veins up past valves (1) which close (2) to stop backflow. Standing increases the pressure on the valves.

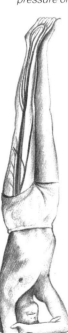

Varicose veins
Pressure from long periods of standing, and insufficiency of the valves in peripheral veins, may cause the blood to run back to the superficial veins. These dilate and twist – a condition we call varicose veins.

Inverted poses
Inverting the body reverses the effect of gravity, resting the valves and vein walls. The blood pours down into head and neck without exertion by the heart. Regular practice prevents and alleviates varicose conditions.

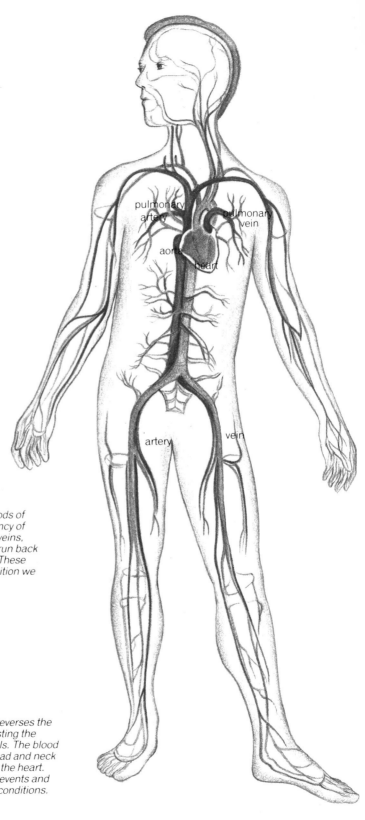

pulmonary artery

pulmonary vein

aorta

heart

artery

vein

The Vital Balance

In any ordinary day, your mind and body handle countless different activities designed to serve your needs, carry out your intentions and ensure your health and survival. The body is the perfect instrument of the mind, responding to every stimulus and command sent out by its messenger systems – the spreading network of nerves and the circulating hormones in the blood. If the nervous system is like a vast, complex telephone exchange, the endocrine (hormonal) system is like the body's climate control and weathercock, preparing you for approaching storms or calm. Both systems supply information and provoke action in response, and between them they regulate every function in your body – its state of arousal or rest, its energy output, and the stability of its internal environment, vital to health. Your emotions both influence, and are influenced by these messengers: if you feel afraid, your body shows the symptoms of fear – faster heartbeat, sweating, dilated pupils and so on; if your body is producing these symptoms, you will feel afraid.

The most important work of the yoga asanas is in strengthening and purifying the nervous system, particularly the spinal cord and nerve ganglia, as these correspond to the routes of prana in the subtle body. The different asanas systematically stretch and tone all the peripheral nerves, helping to strengthen them and to stabilize neuro-chemical transmission. They also tone the sympathetic and parasympathetic nervous systems, which act in opposition to regulate voluntary and involuntary functions. Active signals from the sympathetic nerves stimulate our response to need or emergency, particularly the "fight or flight" response to stress, while inhibiting the functions controlled by the parasympathetic system, such as the flow of saliva and gastric juices, and the normalisation of pulse and breathing. The asanas also massage and stimulate all the endocrine glands.

If your nervous and endocrine systems are healthy, body and mind will respond positively to demand or threat, and quickly return to normal functioning. But if nervous system and hormonal levels become unbalanced, perpetually sending messages of emergency and overreacting to stress, then exhaustion, hypertension, anxiety and depression, and nervous disorders will result. And if the functions of vital glands are depressed, the body metabolism may be out of balance too, causing obesity, menstrual problems, and ultimately serious disease. Research shows that yoga exercise burns only 0.8 calories per minute, as opposed to 0.9 to 1.0 calories in a resting subject, and up to 14 calories per minute in other types of exercise. Asana practice effectively controls hypertension and anxiety, and restores stress resistance, correct metabolism, and healthy nervous transmission. The gentle yoga exercise can be performed by anyone, even during illness – its health-giving properties are available to all.

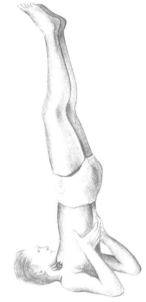

Thyroid and Shoulderstand

Some people seem fireballs of energy, able to eat what they like without putting on weight, while others need a lighter pace and easily gain weight. Such differences are largely due to the thyroid gland in the neck. If it is underactive, the whole body slows down – you feel lethargic and cold, cannot think fast, lose appetite, but still gain weight. If it is overactive, you burn up energy, tend to lose weight, and may be excitable and nervous. A healthy thyroid is vital to well being. In the Shoulderstand, your concentration and circulation are entirely directed to the thyroid, as it is massaged and stimulated, restoring a healthy metabolism.

Glands

All the intricate life functions of body chemistry are regulated by the "ductless" or endocrine glands, secreting their chemical messengers into the blood-stream. Rather like the opposing muscles of the skeletal system, the endocrine system acts on a principle of balance – one hormone stimulates a set of responses, another inhibits it, and all act together in a complex interrelationship with each other, and with the sympathetic nervous system, under the control of the pituitary, and ultimately of the brain and mind. The endocrine system mediates the intimate relationship of body and mind – emotions such as fear or rage, love or grief, both reflect hormonal activity and influence it strongly. A severe shock or tragedy upsets the whole system, and may cause illness. Yoga can restore the system to balance before long term damage is done.

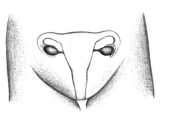

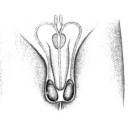

Female sex hormones
The ovaries are the main source of oestrogen, the hormone which regulates the menstrual cycle, pregnancy, breast feeding, and female physical appearance and sexuality. The Backward and Forward Bends massage the womb and ovaries, the Cobra being especially helpful for painful or irregular menstruation.

Male sex hormones
The testes are the main source of the male sex hormone, testosterone. Regular practice of asanas, pranayama and relaxation keeps the male hormones in balance and helps to relieve sexual problems and disorders.

The pituitary gland
This master gland regulates secretion in all the other endocrine glands, and is directly controlled by the brain. The Headstand is the most beneficial asana here.

Thyroid and parathyroid
The thyroid controls the basal metabolic rate, growth, and cell processes. The parathyroid controls calcium and phosphate in the blood. Both are massaged by the Shoulderstand.

Pancreatic and adrenal glands
The secretions of these glands are essential to life, affecting your emotional and physical state strongly. The pancreas produces insulin to regulate blood sugar, and is helped by the Peacock which massages it and the spleen. The adrenal cortex produces sex hormones, and the vital corticosteroids; the medulla secretes adrenalin (also released at sympathetic nerve endings), to arouse the body to "fight or flight". Asanas, relaxation and meditation stabilize stress reactions and adrenalin secretion.

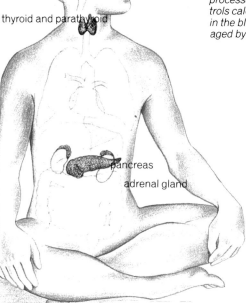

pituitary gland

thyroid and parathyroid

pancreas

adrenal gland

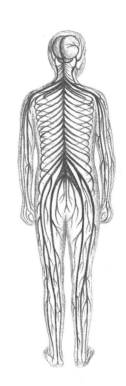

Nerves

A healthy nervous system enables you to meet every event of life with calm and resilience. It keeps all the muscles, organs and tissues of the body working at full efficiency, gives sharper sensory perception, and creates a sense of vitality and energy in your whole being. The nervous system is made up of large numbers of individual cells, or neurones, each with a cell body and long projecting fibres that transmit rapid trains of nerve impulses or signals. Bundles of fibres together form the large nerves, which are stretched and purified by your asanas. By clearing toxins from the tissues, the asanas benefit neurotransmission at the fine nerve endings, and at synapses between nerves. Yoga has been shown to stabilize the response of the nervous system to stress, removing the constant muscular tension produced by repeated alerts from the central nervous system, and calming the involuntary symptoms of threat – racing heart, sweating, anxiety – roused by the sympathetic nervous system.

Peripheral Nervous System
The spinal nerves leave the cord in pairs from either side of each segment, and branch finely to form the peripheral system. The motor (efferent) fibres carry instructions to every muscle, the sensory (afferent) fibres bring in information from every receptor. The autonomous system (sympathetic/parasympathetic) which mediates involuntary functions, also arises from the spine: sympathetic nerve fibres carry major ganglia (control centres), close to the spinal column, which are toned by stretching the spine. Yogis can achieve voluntary influence of the sympathetic system.

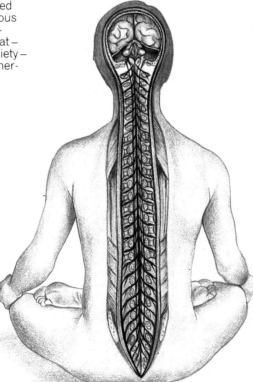

Central Nervous System
The central nervous system is the power house and communications centre of the body. From their deep roots in the cord, the spinal nerves spread out to serve every part of the system. Within the cord, a ceaseless intercommunication takes place, and impulses travel rapidly up and down the sensory and motor fibres, to and from the brain. The asanas work strongly on every part of the spinal column, indirectly stretching the spinal cord, toning the nerve roots and freeing the nerves of any pressure as they emerge from the spinal column.

188

Glossary of Sanskrit Terms

A

Agni Sara *a kriya to massage the digestive organs; agni means fire*
Ahimsa *non-violence; a yama*
Ajna Chakra *the sixth chakra, between the eyebrows*
Akarna Dhanurasana *Shooting Bow*
Anahata Chakra *the fourth chakra, at the heart*
Ananda *bliss*
Anjaneyasana *Crescent Moon; Splits*
Anuloma Viloma *alternate nostril breathing in pranayama*
Apana *the descending breath; a manifestation of prana*
Ardha Matsyendrasana *Half Spinal Twist*
Ardha Padmasana *Half Lotus*
Asana *posture (literally "seat")*
Ashram *a hermitage*
Atman *the Self, Soul, Spirit*

B

Bandha *muscular lock or contraction to control the flow of prana*
Bandha Padmasana *Bound Lotus*
Basti *a kriya for lower colon irrigation*
Bhakti Yoga *the yogic path of devotion*
Bhastrika *a rapid variety of pranayama; bellows breathing*
Bhujangasana *Cobra*
Bija Mantra *seed mantra or Sanskrit letter, denoting the power of a deity or element*
Brahma *in the Hindu Trinity, the Creator*
Brahman *the Absolute*
Brahmari *a variety of pranayama; the "humming" breath*

C

Chakra *one of seven centres of pranic energy*
Chakrasana *Wheel*
Chin Mudra *a hand mudra, linking the thumb and index finger*

D

Dhanurasana *Bow*
Dharana *concentration*
Dhauti *a kriya for cleansing the stomach, by swallowing a cloth*
Dhyana *meditation*

G

Garbhasana *Foetus*
Garuda Asana *Eagle*
Guna *one of the three qualities that make up the whole of the manifest universe or Prakriti*
Guru *a teacher, literally the "remover of darkness"*

H

Halasana *Plough*
Hatha Yoga *practical branch of Raja Yoga, that includes the asanas, pranayama and kriyas; "hatha" means sun and moon*

I

Ida *one of the main nadis, flowing through the left nostril*

J

Jalandhara Bandha *chin lock*
Janu Sirasana *Head to Knee Pose*
Japa *repetition of a mantra*
Jiva *individual soul*
Jnana Yoga *the yogic path of knowledge*

K

Kakasana *Crow*
Kapalabhati *a kriya and pranayama that cleanses the respiratory system*
Kapotha Asana *Pigeon*
Karma *the law of cause and effect; literally "action"*
Karma Yoga *the yogic path of selfless service*
Krishna *an incarnation of Vishnu*
Kriya *a purification practice*
Kukutasana *Cock*
Kundalini *the potential spiritual energy*
Kunjar Kriya *a kriya to clean the stomach*
Kurmasana *Tortoise*

M

Mala *a string of beads, used in japa*
Manas *mind*
Manipura Chakra *the third chakra, at the solar plexus*
Mantra *a sacred syllable, word or phrase, used in meditation*
Matsyasana *Fish*
Matsyendrasana *Spinal Twist*
Maya *illusion*
Mayoorasana *Peacock*
Meru *the largest bead in a mala*
Moola Bandha *anal lock*
Mudra *gesture or posture for controlling prana*
Muladhara Chakra *the first chakra, at the base of the spine*

N

Nadi *nerve channel*
Natarajasana *Lord Nataraja's Pose*
Nauli *a kriya for cleaning the nasal passage*
Nirguna *a type of meditation; literally "without qualities"*
Niyama *one of five observances*

O

Om *the original mantra*
Oordhwapadmasana *Lotus Headstand*

P

Pada Hasthasana *Head to Feet Pose; Hands to Feet Pose*
Padandgushtasana *Tiptoe Pose*
Padmasana *Lotus*
Paschimothanasana *Forward Bend*
Pingala *one of the main nadis, flowing through the right nostril*
Poorna Supta Vajrasana *Diamond*
Prakriti *nature, the manifest universe*
Prana *vital energy, the life force*
Pranayama *regulation of breath, a breathing exercise*
Pratyahara *withdrawal of the senses*
Purusha *spirit*

R

Raja Yoga *the yogic path of meditation*
Rajas *the guna of activity*

S

Saguna *a type of meditation; literally "with qualities"*
Sahasrara Chakra *the seventh and highest chakra, at the crown of the head*
Salabhasana *Locust*
Samadhi *superconsciousness*
Samanu *a variety of pranayama that cleanses the nadis*
Sarvangasana *Shoulderstand*
Satchitananda *existence, knowledge and bliss*
Sattva *the guna of purity*
Sethu Bandhasana *Bridge*
Shakti *the active feminine principle*
Shanti *peace*
Simhasana *Lion Pose*
Sirshasana *Headstand*
Sithali, Sitkari *varieties of pranayama that cool the body*
Siva *in the Hindu Trinity, the Destroyer; the passive male force*
Sukhasana *Easy Pose*
Supta Vajrasana *Kneeling Pose*
Surya *the sun*
Surya Bheda *a variety of pranayama that heals the body*
Surya Namaskar *Sun Salutation*
Sushumna *the main nadi, flowing through the spinal cord*
Sutra *an aphorism, literally "thread"*
Swadhishthana Chakra *the second chakra, at the genitals*
Swami *monk*

T

Tamas *the guna of inertia*
Tratak *steady gazing; a kriya and concentration technique*
Trikonasana *Triangle*

U

Uddiyana Bandha *a lock that brings the diaphragm upward*
Ujjayi *a variety of pranayama*
Uthitha Kurmasana *Balancing Tortoise*

V

Vatayanasana *Wind Relieving Pose*
Vatyanasana *One Knee and Foot Pose*
Vedanta *school of philosophy; literally "the end of knowledge"*
Vedas *the highest authority of all Aryan scriptures, revealed to sages during meditation*
Veerasana *Warrior*
Vishnu *in the Hindu Trinity, the Preserver*
Vishnu Mudra *a hand mudra, used in pranayama*
Vishuddha Chakra *the fifth chakra, at the throat*
Vrikshasana *Handstand*
Vrischikasana *Scorpion*

Y

Yama *one of five restraints*
Yantra *a geometric diagram, used in meditation*
Yoga *union of the individual soul with the Absolute*
Yogi, Yogini *one who practises yoga*

Recommended Reading

Serpent Power Arthur Avalon
Ten Talents Dr and Mrs Frank J. Hurd
Diet for a Small Planet Francis Moore Lappe
Mind, Its Mysteries and Control Swami Sivananda
Sadhana Swami Sivananda
Thought Power Swami Sivananda
Pancadasi Sri Vidyaranya Swami
Complete Illustrated Book of Yoga Swami Vishnu Devananda
Raja Yoga Swami Vivekananda

Index

Sivananda Yoga Vedanta Centres

Ashrams
Sivananda Ashram Yoga Camp HQ
8th Avenue, VAL MORIN
QUE JOT 2RO, CANADA
or P.O. Box 658, Plattsburg
N.Y. 12901
Tel: (819) 322-3226

Sivananda Yoga Ranch Colony
Route 1, Box 228A, WOODBOURNE
NEW YORK, N.Y. 12788
Tel: (914) 434-9242

Sivananda Ashram Yoga Retreat
P.O. Box N7550, NASSAU
BAHAMAS
Tel: (809) 325-5902

Sivananda Yoga Dhanvanthari
Ashram, P.O. Neyyar Dam
Trivandrum Dt., KERALA STATE
INDIA
Tel: 695-576

Sivananda Áshram Yoga Farm
Vrindavan, P.O. Box 795
GRASS VALLEY, CALIFORNIA
CA 95945

Centres
AUSTRALIA
Sivananda Yoga Vedanta Centre
78 Enoggera Terrace, Red Hill
BRISBANE

AUSTRIA
Sivananda Yoga Zentrum
Rechte Wienzeile 29-3-9
VIENNA

CANADA
Sivananda Yoga Vedanta Center
5178 St Lawrence Blvd.
MONTREAL, QUE H2T 1R8
Tel: (514) 279-3545

Sivananda Yoga Vedanta Center
835 Brown Street, QUEBEC CITY
Tel: (418) 843-5563

FRANCE
Centre de Yoga Sivananda
123 Boul. Sebastopol
PARIS
Tel: (33) 261-7749

GERMANY
Sivananda Yoga Zentrum
Steinheilstr. 1, 8 MUNICH 2
Tel: (089) 52-44-76

ISRAEL
Sivananda Yoga Vedanta Centre
4 Yochanan Hasandlar St.
TEL AVIV
Tel: 28-23-20

Sivananda Yoga Centre (affiliated)
Shoshanat Hacarmel 46
HAIFA 34322
Tel: 83625

SPAIN
Association International Sivananda
Yoga Vedanta Centro
C/Juan Bravo 62, 7A, MADRID 6
(01) 402-7467

Centro de Yoga Ananda
(affiliated)
Teresa Herrera 7-1, LA CORUNA
(981) 226-013

Sivananda Yoga Centre
(affiliated)
Joaquin Costa 55, VALENCIA 5
(96) 333-1352

Centro de Yoga de Vigo
Progreso 22-3, VIGO
(89) 227-7321

SWITZERLAND
Centre de Yoga Sivananda
1 Rue de Minoteries, GENEVA
Tel: (22) 28-03-28

URUGUAY
Asociacion de Yoga Sivananda
Acevedo Diaz 1525, 1
MONTEVIDEO
Tel: 49-54-64

UNITED KINGDOM
Sivananda Yoga Vedanta Centre
50 Chepstow Villas, LONDON W11
Tel: 229-7970

UNITED STATES
Sivananda Yoga Vedanta Center
243 West 24th Street, NEW YORK
NY 10011
Tel: (212) 255-4560

Sivananda Yoga Vedanta Center
1929 19th Street N.W.
WASHINGTON D.C. 20009
Tel: (202) 331-9642

Sivananda Yoga Vedanta Center
1246 Bryn Mawr, CHICAGO
ILL 60660
Tel: (312) 878-2468

Sivananda Yoga Vedanta Center
739 N.W. 2nd Ave. FORT
LAUDERDALE
FLORIDA, FLA 33301
Tel: (305) 467-7632

Sivananda Yoga Acres
Rt.4, Box 112, FORT PIERCE
FLORIDA, FLA 33450
Tel: (305) 465-9976

International Sivananda Yoga
Community, 8157 Sunset Blvd.
LOS ANGELES,
CALIFORNIA, CA 90046
Tel: (213) 654-6785 or 650-9452

Authors' Acknowledgements

"Thy right is to work only; but never with its fruits; let not the fruit of action be thy motive, nor let thy attachment be to inaction."
Bhagavad Gita

We should like to thank:
Lucy, who was able to capture an idea, and through her sensitivity, to put magic into the words.
Fausto, who through his perception, was able to recreate the feeling of an asana in colours and capture it on film.
Joss, Chris, Ros, Tony and Dave, who through their combined patience and skill helped to spread the idea.
Hari Markman who gently spread his asanajai.
Mahadev for his selflessness.
Hamsa Patel, Surya Joplin-Waters, and Ben Chissick for spreading their widsom of age.
Sujata Mintz, our Divine Mother.
All the other aspiring Hatha Yogis: Barbara, Parameshwari, Parvati, Chandra, Prem, Cye, Nataraj, Omkar, Danny, Amari, Demian, Zoe and Scott.
Sandra Simmons for your kindness.
Surya Kumari for sharing your knowledge.
Harold Elvin for general advice.
Swami Padmapadananda, Gauri Shankar, Omkar Mintz, and Mark Le Fanu for their expertise.
Dr J.T. Vyas MS, FICS, Dr H. Kulmar MRCP and P. Bardaji MB, NDDO for their medical advice.
Rose, Esther, Bernie and Fred for their patience.
Kanti Devi and Yashoda who gave love where and when it was needed most.
Max, Giorgio, Armando and to Sivadas and the many other nameless Karma Yogis who through their selfless service helped to bring you this idea.

OM TAT SAT

Publisher's Acknowledgments

Gaia would like to extend special thanks to:
Swami Vishnu Devananda for his help and support; Lucy, Fausto, Narayani, Giris, Hari, and the staff of the Sivananda Yoga organization who made the book possible; the illustrators for their skill and hard work; Michael Burman; Peter Carroll; Raj Patel; and the following organizations: E. Gandolfi Ltd, 150 Marylebone High Street, London, W.1 for leotards and tights; Yoga for Health Foundation, Ickwell Bury, Biggleswade, Beds. for yoga mats; Barker's of Kensington; and Pot Pourri.

Illustrators
Lindsay Blow
Felicity Edholm
Elaine Keenan
Tony Kerins
Tony Lodge
Gary Marsh
Sheilagh Noble
Rodney Shackle
David Whelan

Illustration Style
Sheilagh Noble
Rodney Shackle

Typesetting by:
Bookworm Typesetting, Manchester

Reproduction by:
F.E. Burman Ltd., London

Picture Credits
British Museum:
Yogi practising nyasa, p.68
Cliché Musées Nationaux:
Yogi with disciple, p.176
(photo Documentation Photographique de la Réunion des Musées Nationaux)
Mary Evans Picture Library:
Yogi with pet peacock, p.17
A.F. Kersting (photo):
Wheel from the temple of Surya,
Konarak, Orissa, p.18
Ajit Mookerjee:
Statuette of a yogi, p.13
(photo Oriental Museum, Durham)
Ajit Mookerjee:
Subtle body of the yogi, p.81
(photo Thames and Hudson)
Musée Guimet:
Fasting Buddha, p.87
(photo Giraudon)
Harry Oldfield:
Kirlian photograph, p.12
Anne & Bury Peerless (photo):
Siva as a Mahayogi, p.14
Enlightened Buddha, p.87
Sivananda Yoga Life (photo):
H.H. Sri Swami Sivananda, p.20
Victoria & Albert Museum:
The Sage and the King, p.15
(photo Michael Holford)